Lemon Tree Very Healthy Cookbook

ZESTFUL RECIPES WITH JUST THE RIGHT TWIST OF LEMON

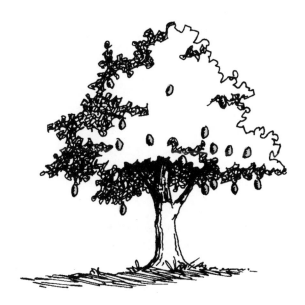

Sunny Baker
Michelle Sbraga

Illustrated by John Wincek

Avery Publishing Group

Garden City Park, New York

Cover designers: William Gonzalez and Rudy Shur
Cover Art: William Gonzalez
Cover photo: John Strange
Text illustrator: John Wincek
In-house editors: Joanne Abrams and Elaine Will Sparber
Typesetter: Baker & Baker/John and Rhonda Wincek
Printer: Paragon Press, Honesdale, PA

Library of Congress Cataloging-in-Publication Data

Baker, Sunny.
      Lemon tree very healthy cookbook : zestful recipes with just the right
twist of lemon : everything you need to know about lemons in one volume /
Michelle Sbraga, Sunny Baker ; illustrated by John Wincek.
          p.   cm.
      "Over 220 tasty lemon recipes."
      Includes index.
      ISBN 0-89529-626-8
      1. Cookery (Lemons). 2. Lemon. I. Sbraga, Michelle. II. Title.
TX813.L4S27   1994
641.6'4334—dc20   94-19239
                                                     CIP

10 9 8 7 6 5 4 3 2 1

Contents

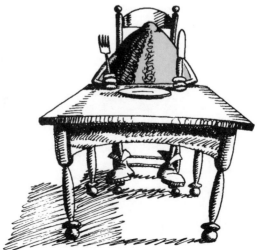

To my mom, Norma Staron, who had the good sense to let me play in the kitchen, and to Kim, who is my best friend, husband, and chief taster.

—Sunny Baker

To my mother, Letitia Gregory, who showed me that the kitchen is a place for adventure, and to my husband, Michael, who is always willing to go along for the ride.

—Michelle Sbraga

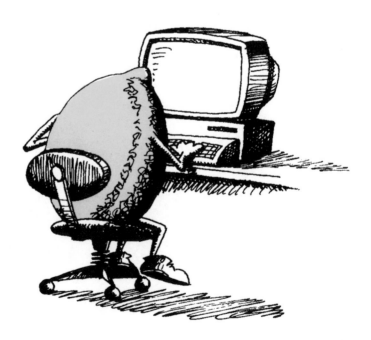

Acknowledgments

Like most books, this one was not a solitary effort. Along with the thousands of lemons that helped us in our quest for the best zesty, tangy, spicy, and healthy recipes, there are many people to thank.

First, our husbands, who never complained about all of the lemons in the kitchen cupboards or on their plates—we love you for trying every experiment. Your good senses of humor kept us going when the experiments turned sour and encouraged us when things were sweet.

Our appreciation also goes to our many friends who gave us guidance and graciously shared their recipes—Patricia Tiffany, Jan Warren Davies, Steve Fullmer, Colette Lejcar, Johnnie Forquer, Kathy Cunningham, Harriet McCallister, Jan Mangelsdorf, Lois Heil, Jean George, and Sunkist Growers. Also, our thanks are extended to the Mesa Public Library, Phoenix Public Library, and Tempe Public Library for their wonderful research facilities and dedicated staffs.

Most of all, we'd like to thank John Wincek, illustrator and friend, who made this book even more delightful with his wonderful taste for whimsy.

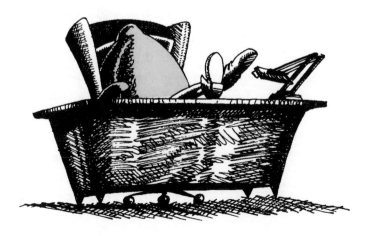

Preface

Fresh lemons—ten for one dollar. The abundant fruit beckons in yellow splendor from roadside stands, produce departments, and backyard trees. You know the lemons are a bargain, but what can you do with so many of them?

While it's true that lemons in season are a good deal across the nation and a central ingredient in healthy, natural cooking, the fruit may be plentiful, but the lemon recipes are not. The recipes are scattered about in various cookbooks and in forgotten files, folders, and drawers—and the potential of the lemon is left unfulfilled. We didn't want any of those golden, prodigious fruits to have such a sour fate, so as self-admitted lemonphiles and proud lemon-tree owners, we decided to put all our lemon recipes together in one place, and *Lemon Tree Very Healthy Cookbook* is the result. We've tried to include everything you need to know about using lemons in recipes. With the information in this book, you will know exactly what to do with all those wonderful yellow bundles. Also, keep your eyes peeled for the "Lemonaids" that we have sprinkled throughout the book. They are filled with dozens of handy lemon tips and bits of information about using our favorite fruit around the house.

Optimists propose, "When life gives you lemons, make lemonade." This is a great suggestion as far as it goes, but there are a thousand other things to make when luscious lemons are bountiful. *Lemon Tree Very Healthy Cookbook* not only tells you exactly what to do with the lemons and lemon-flavored herbs in your life, it puts the information all in one place. Before finishing this book, you will realize that those ten lemons you bought probably won't get you through a full week! You'll agree with us that no healthy kitchen is complete without fresh lemons tucked away somewhere.

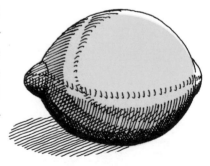

Chapter 1

The Sweet Story of Lemons

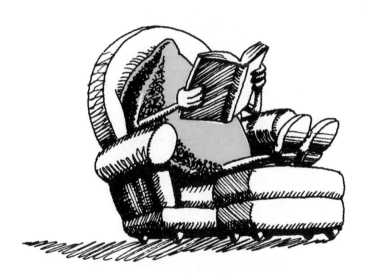

The lemon holds a treasured place in citrus lore. Following in the footsteps of conquering armies and invading hordes, the lemon brought civilization shelter, freedom from sickness, and a tangy twist for iced tea to all corners of the globe. The story of the lemon is not the simple story of a solitary fruit. It is the saga of an entire citrus family, and a vast crowd of related lemony herbs, all with the power to turn ordinary fare into an eating adventure.

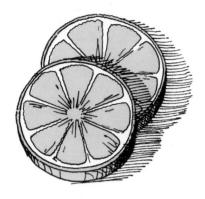

Lemons and Healthy Meals—
A Natural Pair

art, refreshing, inviting, summery, zesty, tingly—these are the words that come to mind when we hear the word *lemon.* But *healthy?*

Lemons are as important as fresh vegetables and herbs are in today's health-conscious cooking. Like all other citrus fruits, lemons are high in ascorbic acid (Vitamin C), which is essential to our health. While most mammals can synthesize their own ascorbic acid internally, humans must obtain it from food sources. Because our bodies don't store this necessary vitamin, we must replenish it every day.

Scurvy, once the scourge of the Seven Seas, is the result of a severe lack of Vitamin C. Some of the early signs of a Vitamin C deficiency include weight loss, bleeding gums, weakness, lassitude, irritability, and easy bruising.

Vitamin C not only fends off scurvy, but it also is necessary for tissue growth and repair. It is vitally important for the proper formation of teeth and bones, and it helps us resist infection by supporting the immune system. It also enhances the body's absorption of iron from grains, fruits, and vegetables. Recent medical research, though not definitive, indicates that high doses of Vitamin C supplements and plentiful amounts of certain foods rich in Vitamin C may help protect against cancer and reduce the risk of heart disease. It's an amazing vitamin—and lemons have lots of it. Since Vitamin C is unstable and is easily destroyed by oxygen, alkalis, and high temperatures, it is important that we include natural, fresh sources of Vitamin C in our diet—and, again, lemons offer a perfect solution.

The government's daily recommended dietary allowance (RDA) of Vitamin C for anyone over the age of fifteen is 60 milligrams. While it is certainly important to meet the recommended dietary allowance of Vitamin C, the RDA is actually the absolute minimum amount you must take to avoid deficiency problems. You can optimize your health by surpassing the RDA and taking between 500 and 5,000 milligrams, depending upon your state of health, according to Shari Lieberman and Nancy Bruning in *The Real Vitamin and Mineral Book* (Garden City Park, NY: Avery Publishing Group, 1990). Temporarily raising your Vitamin C intake during times of stress or infection can help to speed your recovery. However, you should first confirm any major change of intake with your doctor to be sure it doesn't conflict with a prescribed treatment.

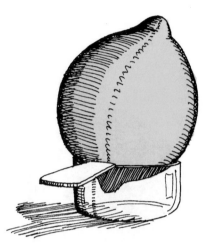

One cup of fresh lemon juice provides 112 milligrams of ascorbic acid. It also has 344 milligrams of potassium (an important salt that balances sodium in the blood system) and only 60 calories. And all of this is wrapped up in a pretty yellow package that fits right in the palm of your hand.

While you might not go out of your way to drink a cup of pure lemon juice every day, or to eat a raw lemon (39 milligrams of ascorbic acid, 102 milligrams of potassium, 2 milligrams of sodium, and only 20 calories), the daily use of lemons and their juice in your cooking will help you obtain the necessary amount of Vitamin C—naturally and deliciously.

More Than Vitamin C to Offer

L emons provide benefits other than Vitamin C as well. They are very low in calories and contain absolutely no fat. The tangy flavor of lemons adds a sophisticated dimension to main dishes and desserts—one that minimizes the need for salt and oil in many recipes. This adds up to healthier foods with no sacrifice of flavor.

As most of us now know, the less salt used, the better. There is no established RDA for salt, but it is estimated that an adequate adult intake ranges from 1,100 to 3,300 milligrams of sodium daily, depending on physical activity and personal requirements. There are 1,938 milligrams of sodium in one teaspoon of ordinary table or sea salt. (Sea salt, though still mostly sodium, is a somewhat better ingredient than ordinary processed table salt because it contains important trace minerals that facilitate the assimilation of vitamins and balanced blood chemistry. For this reason, we suggest that you use sea salt in your shaker if you must have salt at the table.)

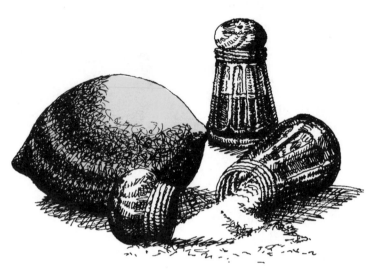

Our bodies need sodium to help maintain a proper balance of water. Too much salt, though, increases the body's retention of water. Salt, as sodium chloride and related chemical compounds, is contained in many of the foods we eat, giving us more than enough salt without the need to add more.

One way to get around adding more salt during cooking is to add lemon juice, lemon zest, or the whole fruit by itself or in combination with herbs and spices. When a dish "needs a little something," many times it has been overcooked, and the taste we're looking for is usually that of an acid—not salt. With its tart, fresh taste, lemon fits the bill perfectly.

At our dinner parties, we put lemon slices on the guests' plates as a garnish. This dresses up the presentation and encourages people to squeeze a little lemon juice on their food instead of pouring on the salt. For those who feel the urge to shake a little something on their food, we often provide a little dish of *gremolata* to substitute for salt. (Our simple gremolata recipe can be found on page 228.) The gremolata adds plenty of extra tang to any main dish—and no extra salt or calories.

When switching over to a healthier lifestyle, people usually eat more salads. Salads of greens or fruit are, indeed, very healthy. But the oil-based dressings that cover the salads are relatively high in fat. Even olive oil, which is rich in the healthier monounsaturated fats, is still a fat. Although there is growing evidence that reducing the fat in your diet is an important component of a healthy lifestyle, it's tough to forego the dressings and eat naked greens. Fortunately, lemon juice provides a clean, crisp base for salad dressings with enough body and spark to minimize or even eliminate the need for oil. Lemon juice perks up a boring salad with its tangy flavor, and it doesn't leave the heavy, cloying after-taste that is so common to bottled dressings.

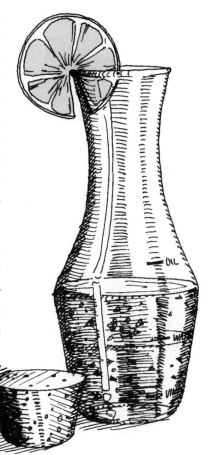

When putting together the dressing for your next salad, reach for a lemon. On page 221, we provide a basic recipe for Light Lemon Vinaigrette, a mixture that can be used as a general-purpose marinade or as a dressing on almost any salad or vegetable. This simple dressing can be substituted for the higher-calorie oil-based vinaigrettes that are frequently called for in gourmet recipes. We provide many other lemon-based sauces and dressings in this book that are every bit as tasty as their oil-heavy cousins and much lower in calories and fat.

For people who occasionally want an oil-based dressing, we've included some recipes for those as well, but we advise you to use them sparingly. When we want a quick lemon-and-oil dressing, we simply squeeze the juice of half a lemon on a mass of fresh greens and then toss in just a few dribbles of high-quality virgin olive oil. Be sure to use the oil in moderation. After all, some oil in the diet is a good thing—but like salt, a little goes a long way.

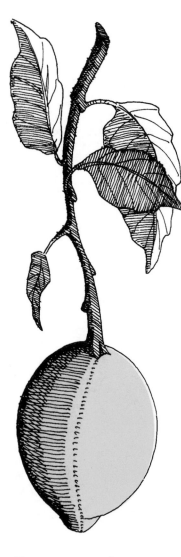

E U R E K A   L E M O N

Butter is definitely not the fat of choice in healthy living. Always remember to reach for a lemon instead of butter when serving vegetables. Besides being much better for you than butter is, a spritz of lemon juice will bring out the full flavor of vegetables. Even so, zapping vegetables with pure lemon juice all the time can be just as boring as putting a pat of butter or margarine on them. So mix the lemon juice with fresh or dried herbs for even more flavor and a little change of pace. Now if you find you still absolutely must have just a little bit of fat on the vegetables to go with the lemon (we recommend soy margarine), the amount you use will very likely be reduced. With lemon on your side, you might even find yourself losing your taste for fat altogether.

The Incredible, Versatile Lemon

The lemon is delightfully versatile. Lemon preserves, decorates, and enlivens our foods. Lemon brings out the flavor in other foods while providing a unique taste of its own. Lemon's piquant flavor pleases our palates in a main dish, brightens a sauce, and livens up a marinade. Lemon slices and twists add a festive finish to an ordinary presentation. Lemon juice quenches our thirst in soothing teas and satisfying punches. If we occasionally reward ourselves with a sweet treat, lemon pies and tarts wait to satisfy our fancies.

Lemons serve us outside the kitchen as well. Lemon can be dried in potpourris to fill the air with the scent of spring freshness. The juice is a soothing tonic and exfoliant for the skin and can be made into a wonderful conditioner for the hair. Lemon oil keeps our wood furniture like new. As an ingredient in a body splash used after a shower or bath, lemon refreshes the skin and tightens the pores.

In this book, you'll find these and many more uses for lemons. From breakfast to bath, we'll introduce you to literally hundreds of ways to enjoy the mighty lemon. Go ahead, put a little sunshine in your life. Use more lemons!

Once Upon a Time . . .

L emon trees like ours thrive in backyards and porch gardens all across America, but they are most commonly seen in California, Arizona, and Florida. Lemon trees are thought to have originated in Southeast Asia or northwest India near the Himalayas. Archaeologists discovered tomb paintings in the Valley of the Kings which prove that the Egyptians had lemons. The Greeks grew lemon trees alongside their revered olive trees. The Romans took lemons from the Greeks and introduced them to Italy between 100 and 200 A.D. After 568, gardens containing lemon and orange trees were destroyed by the invading Lombards, and the trees died out. By 700, lemon trees were being cultivated in Egypt and Iraq. Around 1100, they were introduced in China. The Arabs took lemon trees into Spain around 1150, and the Crusaders returning from Palestine continued the distribution of the trees in Europe.

In 1493, lemon trees were planted for the first time in Haiti by Christopher Columbus. By 1579, groves of lemons could be found in St. Augustine, Florida, where they flourished up until 1894, when a severe cold spell destroyed the groves. To this day, Florida grows a minimal amount of lemons compared with other citrus fruit crops because of those lost groves.

Spanish missionaries carried lemons into California during the 1700s, but these trees didn't flourish in the climate. The Lisbon lemon was introduced in 1874, and it revolutionized the growth of lemons in the American West. This lemon is considered the best variety for dry, warm inland areas. In 1878, the Eureka lemon was introduced, and today, it is considered the best variety for cool coastal areas.

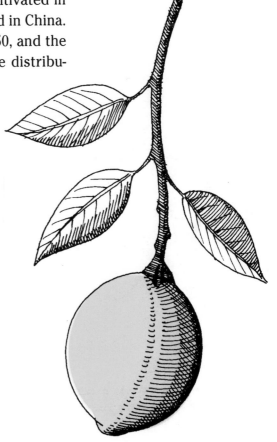

MEYER LEMON

The first commercial orchards in the United States were planted in the late 1800s. Today, the United States raises over 800,000 tons of lemons annually, with California harvesting about 80 percent of the total crop. Arizona is the second biggest producer of lemons in the country. Approximately half of the total United States crop is processed into juice and oil, while the other half is sold as fruit.

Lemon trees now grow all over the world, doing particularly well in semi-arid climates with light rainfall and low humidity. Along with the western United States, Italy, Spain, and Greece are the leading lemon producers, accounting for over half the world's annual harvest of more than 3.5 million tons.

The Care and Feeding of Lemons

If you are lucky, you have a bounty of fresh lemons hanging off a tree in your backyard or in a pot on the porch. A lemon tree can be just as important to a good cook as a windowsill herb garden. If you aren't lucky enough to have your own lemon tree, think about planting one. If you don't enjoy the weather needed to grow citrus fruits, or if you lack the room required for a full-sized tree, consider one of the smaller indoor or porch varieties.

In the United States, lemon trees can be grown almost anywhere. Upstate New York and the plains of Wyoming may not boast lemon orchards, but even there, a lemon tree in a pot on the back porch will give you access to fresh lemons almost year-round. Just bring the pot indoors during the winter freeze. You will be able to breakfast under your lemon tree even when the snow is knee-deep outside.

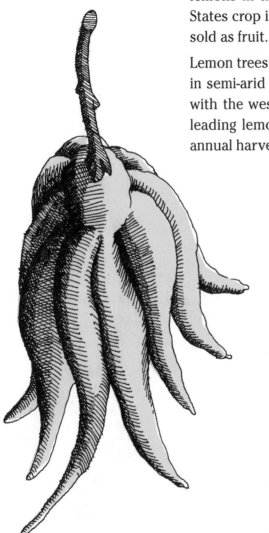

BUDDHA'S HAND

A lemon tree in bloom is enchanting as well as fragrant. Full-sized lemon trees can grow up to twenty-five feet tall. Their pale green leaves are long and pointed, and the branches of some varieties are covered with thorns. (It's a good idea to wear gloves when you're picking lemons from an orchard-sized Lisbon or Ponderosa lemon tree—their branches are full of thorns.) A lemon tree can produce large fragrant blooms almost year-round and often has blossoms and mature fruit at the same time. Although the fruit can be picked from six to ten times a year, lemon trees usually offer major harvests at two times—late summer and mid-winter.

Lemons on the branch take about seven to eight months to ripen. Young trees start bearing fruit as early as three years of age. As the contented owners of backyard lemon trees, we sometimes feel as if our mature trees produce about a million lemons a year. Yes, a slight exaggeration—a mature orchard tree actually produces only about 1,500 lemons a year, and a backyard tree somewhat less. But before we had all of our recipes in hand, it really *seemed* like a million pieces of fruit.

All in the Family

The *citrus limon* of the *Rutaceae* family, more commonly known as the lemon, is a member of the genus *Citrus.* Of the several varieties of lemons grown in the United States, the most prevalent are the Eureka and the Lisbon. The Eureka is a highly acidic, medium-sized variety of lemon. It is the most common commercial lemon. Its nearly thornless tree produces fruit all year in coastal regions and twice a year inland. These trees are very sensitive to cold, insects, and improper handling. Eurekas are best when picked ripe from the tree.

The Lisbon lemon is a highly acidic, medium-sized variety thought to have been developed in Spain. More tolerant of cold than other lemons are, the Lisbon prefers desert and inland areas. This tree has lush foliage and razor-sharp thorns. Lisbons, best when picked ripe from the tree, lose acidity when left on the branch too long.

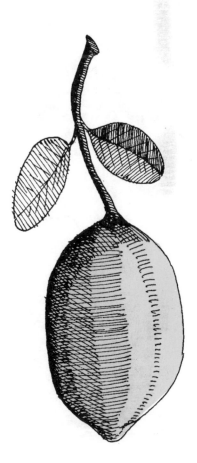

CITRON

The Meyer and Improved Meyer lemon trees have a pale orange fruit. These medium-sized, juicy, and slightly sweet lemons are thought to be hybrids of a lemon and an orange. The hardy, nearly thornless trees, popular in California, are used for hedges and work well in containers. Blooming year-round, Meyers can be left on the tree after maturing. The Meyer varieties are considered sweet lemons. In fact, they do not contain more sugar than other varieties, but simply produce less acid.

The Ponderosa lemon is another hybrid, this time between a lemon and a citron. The thorny tree produces grapefruit-sized, acidic, juicy fruit. Ponderosas have very thick skins and are frost-sensitive. Like the Meyers, these lemon trees can be used for hedges or grown in containers. Blooming all year long, Ponderosas can also be left on the tree after maturity.

The fruit of the Rough lemon tree is not juicy. For this reason, the Rough lemon is used mainly as an ornamental tree and for rootstock. Most Florida orange trees are grown on the Rough lemon rootstock.

Other lemon varieties include the Villafranca, Everbearing, Genoa, Limonera, Monroe, Otaheite, Sicily, Prior, Frost, Nucellar, and Rosenberger. There is also a variety called the Sweet lemon, but it is seldom grown because, ironically, it is not very flavorful.

Citrons are a large, thick-skinned fruit resembling lemons. The trees are sometimes grown as novelties or for Jewish ceremonies. The Etrog is the most commonly planted citron, but the fingered citron known as Buddha's Hand has a more unusual shape. Citrons basically resemble lemons in their cooking characteristics and flavor, except that they offer almost no juice. The Buddha's Hand is almost entirely ornamental, but the Etrog can be used for its zest. The rind is often dried for use in fruitcakes and fragrant potpourris.

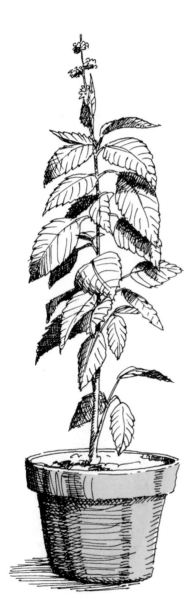

L E M O N   B A L M

How to Love Your Lemon Tree

Truth be told, growing your own lemon tree in those western and southern states that are hot and humid is fairly easy. While the trees can be grown from seedlings, this method requires years of love, patience, and nurturing before a tree produces fruit. But nursery or mail-order trees can bear fruit as little as one year after planting. Except during the winter, lemon trees produce beautiful large white fragrant flowers. Some trees bear fruit for as long as fifty years.

Lemon trees are relatively easy to care for. Plant your tree after the last frost of the season in well-drained soil. With regular watering, fertilizing, and some TLC, you will have many months of fresh lemon enjoyment each year. Keep in mind, though, that neglect can cause mites, thrips, scale insects, or whiteflies, and that trees in poorly drained soil can suffer from root or tree cankers.

While trees grow faster and produce juicier fruit in hot, humid climates, lemon trees are susceptible to sunburn and windburn. Especially in arid climates, slight shade may be required during the summer months, and tree trunks and all exposed branches should be painted with a whitewash.

Cold temperatures are also a problem. Lemon trees are highly susceptible to frost. Lemon fruit can be harmed in as little as thirty minutes in temperatures of 29°F. If frost is a problem in your area, plant your trees in a sunny spot in the yard. The Lisbon is the most cold-tolerant variety of lemon and is most commonly grown in marginal citrus regions. During the occasional frost, the tree can be covered. If frost is a frequent problem, a commercially available "tree tent" should be used and warmed with lights to protect the tree.

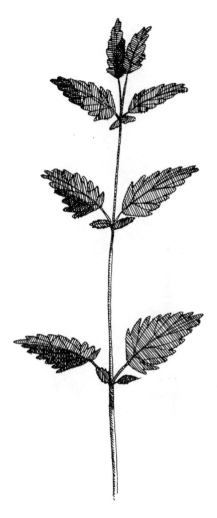

L E M O N   C A T N I P

How to Care for Your Container Tree

Unfortunately, most of the country does not have the best climate for growing lemon trees. But lemon lovers

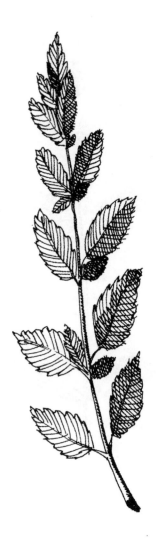

LEMON MINT

need not despair. Lemon trees can easily be grown in containers so that lemonphiles everywhere can revel in the golden fruit. Containers can be placed in the garden or on the back porch during the summer and moved inside during the harsh winter. Imagine picking a lemon off your tree while there are six feet of snow on the ground! Even if you live in citrus country, poor soil or inappropriate drainage may make container trees preferable to backyard varieties.

Container trees need to be planted in good quality potting soil and watered and fertilized frequently. When kept indoors, potted lemon trees need a large sunny window and high humidity. Small trees especially enjoy a bright kitchen window near the steam from the sink. Dry heat will send the trees into shock, usually causing them to drop their leaves. Misting indoor trees with a fine water spray or using a humidifier will help, as will keeping them well away from household heating vents.

Move your container lemon trees indoors or outdoors gradually. By slowly increasing or decreasing their time out of the sun, you'll help the trees adapt to the change in sun levels.

The Lemon-Flavored Herbs

Beyond the fruit, there is another way to get all the lemon flavor we crave. The herb world contains several lemon-scented and lemon-flavored plants that can be used to add new spark to many recipes. Because each has its own lemony nuance, it is not recommended that the herbs be used with too much fresh lemon juice or peel. It will become difficult to know which of your "lemons" you are tasting.

Lemon Balm *(Melissa officinalis)* is an easily grown perennial that stands up to three feet high and comes back dependably year after year. The plants like full sun with midday shade and a moist soil and can be grown indoors. Uses for this herb with a minty-lemon taste go back to antiquity. The ancient

Greeks used it medicinally over 2,000 years ago, and it was sacred to the temple of Diana. Fresh leaves can be finely chopped into vinegars, salads, sauces, mayonnaise, jellies, desserts, and fruit drinks. Dried leaves make a wonderful caffeine-free herb tea. Also try using the dried leaves in potpourris and pillows for a fresh lemon fragrance. Or infuse the leaves and use as a facial steam or as a rinse for oily hair.

Lemon Basil *(Ocimum basilicum citriodorum)* is an annual that grows to a height of eighteen inches and likes full sun. With lighter green leaves than its basil cousins, lemon basil is used in soups, salads, and fish, and as a flavoring for vinegar. It's also popular for use in potpourris.

Lemon Catnip *(Nepeta cataria citriodora)* is a hardy perennial that grows up to three feet tall in full sun or light shade. With a refreshing citrus scent, lemon catnip can be used, fresh or dried, in tea or in salad when young. Like regular catnip, this variety is reputed to have slightly sedative and stomach-calming properties, and it will probably attract the neighborhood cats.

Lemon Mint *(Monarda citriodora)* has a distinctive lemony fragrance. Attaining a height of two feet, this annual herb needs sun with partial shade. Its leaf can be used in hot or iced teas, and in salads and on vegetables.

Orange Mint *(Monarda piperita)* is also called Citrus Mint or Bergamot Mint. With grass-green leaves and lavender flowers, this herb grows to eighteen inches in height and has a wonderful lemon-orange scent. Use it in teas and punches, as a room deodorizer, and in the bath. As with all mint varieties, orange mint and lemon mint are best when fresh.

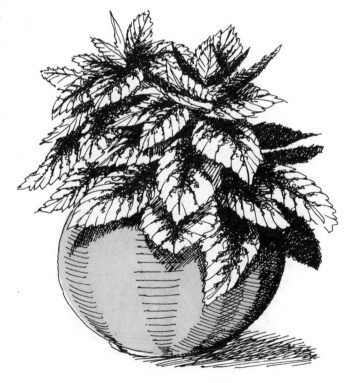

LEMON BALM

Lemon Thyme *(Thymus citriodorus)* is one of over 400 varieties of thyme. It grows to twelve inches in height and likes full sun. It is sometimes better to start a plant from nursery stock than from seed, as lemon thyme can be difficult to get started. Lemon thyme's heavenly lemon flavor is wonderful in teas, eggs, lemon sauces, and cookies.

Lemon Verbena *(Aloysia triphylla)* is a native of South America that loves full sun. It grows from two to fifteen feet tall, depending on the climate. Hotter climates yield taller plants. Lemon verbena is frost-sensitive and must be brought indoors during the winter. The leaves give off a sharp lemony fragrance when rubbed together or broken. This plant offers the truest taste of the lemon-flavored herbs, though it is more subtle than lemon itself. The herb dries well, but the flavor intensifies with drying. Lemon verbena tea with honey is a popular drink called Vervein in France and Herba Louisa Tea in Spain. Lemon verbena can also be used in muffins, jellies, ice milk, and vinegars. Its clean lemon scent is wonderful in herbal pillows and potpourris. You can also add it to your bath water or put it in finger bowls on the dinner table.

Lemongrass *(Cymbopogon citratus)* is used extensively in Southeast-Asian cooking. A tender perennial grass, it grows up to six feet tall in the tropics. While a bit temperamental, it can be grown in the hot or humid climates of the southern and western United States. Look for plants in mail-order nursery catalogues. Most Asian food stores carry lemongrass fresh, frozen, dried, or powdered. Use powdered lemongrass only in extreme emergencies. A better substitute is one and a half

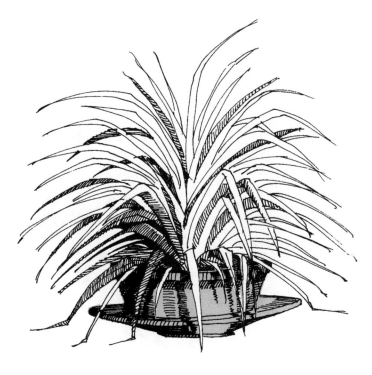

LEMONGRASS

teaspoons of freshly grated lemon zest for each stalk of lemongrass specified. Use lemongrass in tea with cloves, and add it to your soups, salads, and stews. Try using it in potpourris for added fragrance. Lemongrass oil can be used to scent bath water.

Scented Geraniums *(Pelargonium)* come in two lemon scents—Lemon Crispum and Rose-Lemon. These plants grow from one to three feet tall. They take well to containers and make excellent house plants. As tender perennials, scented geraniums prefer sunny, well-ventilated areas and are very frost-sensitive. Used fresh or dried, the leaves retain their lemony scent and can be chopped and added to sauces, jellies, jams, sugar, syrups, and vinegars. The geranium leaf can also be used as a fragrance in potpourris and herbal pillows.

Lemon Marigold is a rare member of the marigold family. An annual, the plant grows six to eight inches high. This plant has petite yellow-orange lemon-scented flowers and a lacy foliage. It cannot be eaten and is grown solely for its lemony fragrance and ornamental qualities.

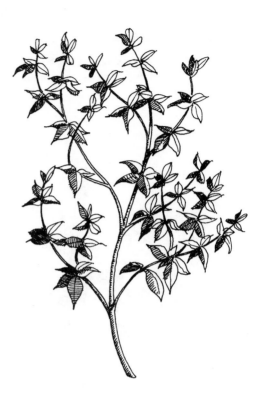

L E M O N   T H Y M E

While dried herbs are fine in most cases, we prefer fresh herbs in our recipes. Unfortunately, lemon-flavored herbs are in short supply in retail markets. But most are easy to grow wherever you live. Visit your local nursery for seed packets and potted plants. Decorate your windowsills and porches with lemon-scented herbs if you don't have the room for a garden. Drying them for your own use will ensure a supply whenever the lemon craving hits.

Lemons will provide you with all manner of health benefits as they liven up your recipes and delight your taste buds. Whether you decide to plant herbs, a tree in a pot, or even a mini-orchard in your backyard, you should have lots of fresh lemons in your life.

Quick Guide to the Lemon-Flavored Herbs

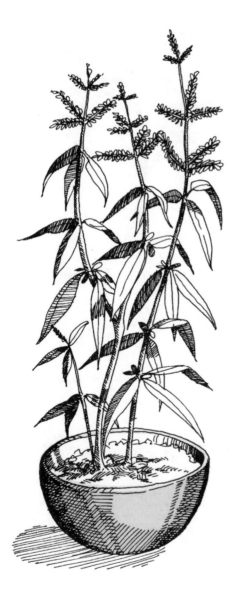

LEMON VERBENA

HERB	CHARACTERISTICS
Lemon Balm	Minty lemon taste. Perennial. Grows up to 3 feet tall.
Lemon Basil	Lighter green leaves than ordinary basil. Annual. Grows up to 18 inches tall.
Lemon Catnip	Citrus scent. Slight sedative and stomach-calming effects. Perennial. Grows up to 3 feet tall.
Lemon Mint	Distinctive minty lemon scent. Annual. Grows up to 2 feet tall.
Orange Mint	Minty lemon-orange scent. Grass-green leaves and lavender flowers. Annual. Grows up to 18 inches tall.
Lemon Thyme	Lemony scent. Grows up to 12 inches tall.
Lemon Verbena	Sharp lemon scent when broken or rubbed. Truest lemon taste of all herbs. Grows from 2 to 15 feet tall.
Lemongrass	Perennial. Grows up to 6 feet tall in tropical climates.
Scented Geraniums	Two scents—Lemon Crispum and Rose-Lemon. Perennials. Grow from 1 to 3 feet tall.
Lemon Marigold	Petite yellow-orange single flowers with lemon scent. Annual. Grows up to 8 inches tall.

GROWING CONDITIONS	CULINARY USES	OTHER USES
Prefers full sun with midday shade and moist soil. Can be grown indoors.	Use in vinegars, salads, sauces, desserts, and fruit drinks. Dry some for teas.	Use in potpourris and herbal pillows. Infuse leaves and use for facial steam or as rinse for oily hair.
Prefers full sun. Can be grown indoors.	Use in soups, salads, fish, and vinegars.	Use in potpourris.
Prefers full sun or light shade.	Use in salads and teas.	Use for cats.
Prefers sun with partial shade.	Use in salads, vegetables, and hot or iced teas.	Use in bath water, as a room deodorizer, and in potpourris.
Prefers sun with partial shade.	Use in teas and punches.	Use in bath water and potpourris.
Prefers full sun. Often easier to start from nursery stock than from seed.	Use in teas, cookies, lemon sauces, and egg dishes.	Use in potpourris.
Prefers full sun. Hotter climates yield taller plants. Frost-sensitive.	Use in teas, muffins, jellies, ice milk, and vinegars.	Use in bath water, finger bowls, herbal pillows, and potpourris.
Prefers full sun and light shade; hot and humid climates. Temperamental.	Use in teas, soups, salads, and stews. Used extensively in Southeast-Asian cooking.	Use in potpourris. Use oil in bath water. Use tea as facial cleanser for oily skin.
Prefer full sun. Frost-sensitive. Take well to containers; make excellent house plants.	Use in sauces, jellies, jams, syrups, and vinegars.	Use flowers for decoration. Use leaves in potpourris and herbal pillows.
Prefers full sun to light shade.	Cannot be eaten.	Use flowers for decoration and fragrance.

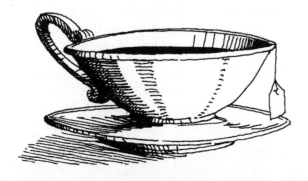

Chapter 2

How to Use Lemons and the Recipes

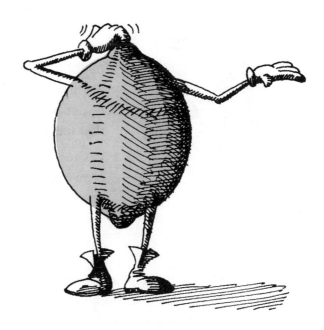

So, you have a basket full of lemons, a willing pair of hands, and an all too eager stomach. What's next? How do you choose, and how do you use, those sunny citrus treasures? If you're ready to try a healthier way of cooking, read on to find out how to get the most from that potential pot of gold.

Preparing Lemons and Their Juices

emons are easy to choose, use, and save. They are as simple to handle as they are zippy in taste. The following pages should answer most of the questions you may have about choosing and using these little yellow gems.

In commercial groves, lemons are picked by size rather than ripeness, and they are usually green when harvested. Why? The earlier lemons are picked after obtaining sufficient size and juiciness, the more acidic they are and the longer they can be safely stored.

When picking lemons from your tree or off the grocer's shelf, look for fruit that is fully yellow. Lemons with green on the

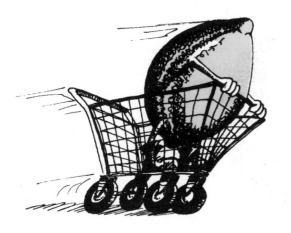

rind will be more acidic and have less flavor. Also be aware that a thick, rough, or pebbly rind is a sign of low juice content. So choose lemons with rinds that are lightly pebbled and thin, and try to find fruit that feels heavy for its size.

If they are available, buy organically grown, pesticide-free lemons—and other produce in general. Organic fruits and vegetables are typically more flavorful than their conventionally processed cousins. Since most of the chemicals end up on the skin, buying pesticide-free lemons is especially important when your recipe calls for lemon zest. If you don't have your own tree and can't find organic produce, be sure to thoroughly rinse your lemons, and your other fruits and vegetables, under cold running water.

Storing Your Lemons

emons should be stored in an airy basket if they will be used within a few days. If left on the counter too long, they may dry up or develop an "off" flavor. Stored in the refrigerator in a plastic bag, they can be kept for up to three weeks without losing any of their tart lemony goodness.

Preserving and Freezing Leftover Lemons

Even devoted lemonphiles can have trouble using up a bountiful harvest. Sometimes there are simply too many lemons on a tree to consume. If you've given the yellow bundles to friends and neighbors and still have hundreds left, try preserving the lemons and juice instead of throwing them away.

Lemons can be stored almost indefinitely when preserved in salt. In a book that emphasizes the use of lemons in place of salt, it is almost comical to suggest that lemons can be preserved with the substance. But it's true. Preserved in this manner (as explained in the recipe for Moroccan Preserved Lemons on page 246), lemons can be kept for about a year. Then, when you want to add lemon flavor to a dish, you can use only the peel—rinsing it well, to eliminate the salt—and discard the pulp. Or you can add the pulp in small quantities to soups and dressings for a bit of tang.

Of course, there's nothing better than fresh lemon juice in your recipes, but it may not always be available. One of the most popular ways to preserve lemon juice is to freeze it in ice trays. The frozen cubes can then be stored in a freezer bag. A bag of frozen lemon-juice cubes is a bag of gold to a cook—and the frozen juice is almost as good as fresh squeezed and certainly an improvement over prepackaged, preserved juices.

Whole lemons can also be frozen. They become very soft when thawed and the juice is easily extracted. Thawed lemons can also be sliced and used in beverages, although they will be somewhat mushy.

While there is nothing wrong with freezing juice or whole fruit, note that the taste will be slightly different from that of

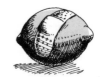

Lemonaid

Never use old, dry lemons in recipes— their taste has turned metallic. Instead, use old lemons and their hulls with some kosher salt to shine up copper. Look for other Lemonaid ideas like this one throughout the book.

fresh lemons. Frozen juice is best used in recipes where it will be cooked, as in stews or soups. For salads and beverages, reach for a fresh lemon whenever possible. Don't even bother with the commercially bottled, reconstituted juice that is preserved with sodium benzoate—it lacks flavor, subtlety, and vitamins.

Getting the Juice Out

Extracting lemon juice for recipes or freezing can be done several ways. Holding a lemon half in your hand and twisting a large fork in the lemon while squeezing the hull is one way. Though this method doesn't always release all the juice, it's fast and simple when you're in a hurry. The juice can simply be filtered through the fingers to catch the pits.

There are also wooden, cone-shaped lemon reamers that fit snugly in the lemon half. These extract all the juice right down to the pith (the white part).

If you're going to extract juice for freezing from a large number of lemons, use a juicer, as it will remove the most liquid gold from your small yellow treasures. There are several good citrus juicers available for under $30 in discount stores.

If a recipe calls for a teaspoon or two of juice and you don't want to cut a whole lemon, use a faucet, which is available in most well-stocked gourmet shops. A faucet turns the lemon into its own bottle. Twist the piece into the lemon, squeeze out the required juice, and snap on the cap. With a faucet in place, you can use the lemon again and again, as needed.

While lemons keep longer in the refrigerator, warm lemons yield more juice. It may be hard, though, to remember to remove the day's lemons from the refrigerator in the morning. In a pinch, put the lemons in the microwave for twenty to thirty seconds, or try soaking them in hot water for ten minutes. If the lemons are already at room temperature, placing them in hot water for a minute or two will make them yield even more juice. Rolling the whole fruit on a countertop a few times will also make it easier to squeeze.

Zesting a Lemon

Whether you call it the skin, peel, zest, or rind, this is where the lemon's flavorful oils are located. Zest is the outermost layer of skin on citrus fruit and contains the most aromatic oils. We always refer to the very outside of the lemon peel as zest to differentiate it from the entire peel, which includes the white pith.

As in everything else, there is more than one way to skin a lemon to get its zest. One way is to use a hand grater. Another way is to use a vegetable peeler, which will take the zest off in larger pieces that may have to be chopped into slivers before being added to a recipe. A third method uses a zester. A zester works like a vegetable peeler but is smaller and made specifically to remove citrus zest. While the recipes in this book always ask for the grated zest of a lemon, the implement you use to get the zest is up to you. However you remove the zest, be very careful not to remove any of the white pith of the peel. The pith will add a bitter taste to your recipes. Again, if you don't have your own tree and organic lemons are unavailable, be sure to wash your lemons well before you begin.

Get into the habit of grating the zest off every lemon you use before squeezing out the juice. If you don't use the zest in a recipe today, dry it out and you can use it tomorrow. Or just grind the dried peels in a blender and store the ground zest in a glass jar on the counter. The sunny yellow hue will brighten up your kitchen, and the handy jar will give you easy access to this flavorful treasure.

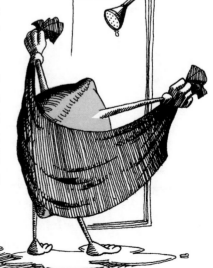

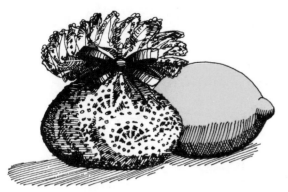

Drying and Preserving Lemon Zest

We keep a little jar of dried lemon zest on the kitchen counter to use in almost every dish—as a garnish to brighten up our culinary creations and to add a bit of zingy flavor. To dry zest, first grate the zest from the lemon while avoiding as much of the bitter pith as possible. Then spread the zest out on a paper towel and allow it to dry overnight. Finally, tie the zest up in a cheesecloth bag and hang it up in the kitchen until the contents have dried. Drying may take up to two days or more, depending on the amount of zest.

Of course, if you live in a wet climate or need some dried zest in a hurry, you can use the oven to expedite the process. Spread the zest on a baking sheet and place the sheet in an oven on the lowest temperature possible until the zest has dried. This takes about three to four hours. Keep a close watch on the zest. If it burns, the flavor will be destroyed. If drying lemon zest for use in potpourris, cut the zest with a knife and leave it in bigger pieces.

Dried zest can be reconstituted and used in recipes calling for fresh zest by placing it in a little water until plump. Lemon zest can also be frozen for later use. Dry it on a baking sheet and freeze it in airtight freezer bags. It can be kept this way for up to six months.

Working With the Acidity of Lemons

The acidic quality of lemons makes lemon juice a natural preservative. You can keep vegetables from discoloring during preparation simply by squeezing on a little lemon juice. Lemon juice added to the water used to steam broccoli or asparagus will keep the vegetables a brilliant green. Added to the water used to prepare cauliflower or rice, lemon juice will allow the foods to retain their natural whiteness.

The acid of lemons has its downside, however. It will react with certain cooking materials, staining the pot, pan, or bowl, or causing it to become pitted. Therefore, it is important to choose nonreactive pots, pans, and bowls when cooking with lemon. Avoid cast iron and aluminum. Instead, use stainless steel, glass, ceramic, or porcelain kitchenware.

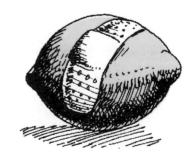

Lemon-Aid Kit

To make your grating, squeezing, and juicing easier, Sunkist Growers, Inc. markets an inexpensive Lemon-Aid Kit. This kit contains a grater, juicer, faucet, two snackers (for peeling), and a recipe booklet. It can be ordered by sending a check for $5.95 payable to Sunkist Lemon-Aid Kit to Sunkist, P. O. Box 4586, Overland Park, Kansas 66204. The kits can also be found in some grocery stores. The kits are a worthwhile investment. We use ours constantly. Sunkist also has a Citrus Hotline to answer your burning lemon questions. You can call (800) 248–7875 weekdays (except holidays) from 10:30 A.M. to 7:00 P.M. (Central Standard Time).

About the Recipes

The recipes in this book support a healthy diet, with little sugar and a minimum of fat. These simple recipes feature a variety of ingredients including tofu, beans, grains, nuts, fresh vegetables, chicken, and fish. The dishes, however, do not include meat. For those who still want some meat and fish in their diets, Chapter 7 presents diverse lemony fish and chicken dishes. We do not offer any recipes using beef or lamb because of the meats' high fat contents. For all of the recipes, we recommend buying only organically grown vegetables, fresh fish, or organically fed free-range chickens. By using only the freshest food available and only ingredients that are organically grown, you can limit your consumption of harmful fertilizers, pesticides, and hormones.

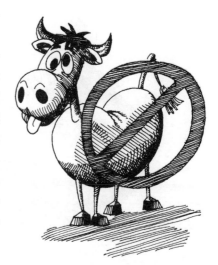

Stocking Your Cupboard

In preparing healthy foods, there are some basic ingredients, beyond lemons, that you'll want to have on hand. These include brown rice, millet, whole grain pastas, whole wheat or other whole grain flours, oat flakes, beans and other dried legumes, extra virgin olive oil, tofu, miso, tahini, soymilk, date sugar, and other foods commonly found in health food stores as well as many well-stocked supermarkets. If you have never used some of these ingredients before, you are in for an adventure of new tastes and textures. Don't let the unusual names of the ingredients scare you. Clear easy-to-follow instructions are provided for guidance. Exotic dishes, and new twists on old favorites, lie in the pages ahead, waiting to delight your senses. Just follow the steps to good eating.

The Sweeteners

Our preference for low-sugar cooking is evident throughout our book. This doesn't mean that every recipe is 100-percent sugar free—we all need a little dessert in our lives once in a while. But you'll find no white, chemically processed sugars in our recipes. You see, processed cane sugar has very little to offer in the way of nutritional value. Therefore, we've banned this abomination from our cupboards. Instead, we use natural products—date sugar, fruit juices, Sucanat, and an occasional bit of honey to sweeten our culinary creations.

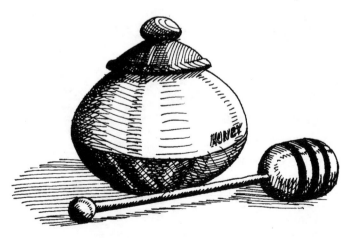

As we've made the transition to healthier cooking over the years, it's been a challenging task to replace the sugar in some of our favorite dessert concoctions. Although the amount of natural sugars has already been reduced in our dessert recipes, it is okay to try a bit less—or more—based upon your preferences. Test different natural sugars in the recipes—date sugar, juices, fruit concentrates, and Sucanat—to get the sweet (or less sweet) taste that you desire.

The Oils

As mentioned earlier, you'll find our recipes to be generally low in fat. We have even provided light versions of lemon standards like lemon pie.

Of course, some oils have healthful benefits. These "good" oils are the unsaturated oils like olive, safflower, canola, and sesame. We use such oils in moderation in our recipes.

When shopping for recipe ingredients, look for oils labeled "unrefined," as these have been mechanically pressed or extracted by low heat. Avoid oils that are generically called "light," especially if they are flavorless and odorless. These oils usually have been chemically treated, bleached, and highly filtered.

In a few of our recipes, we use soy margarine when butter would traditionally be used. Some recipes call for nonfat yogurt or the mock sour cream we make from cottage cheese (see Almost Sour Cream on page 234). Of course, the full-fat varieties of these ingredients can be readily substituted for the nonfat versions, although we don't really recommend doing so.

If you want to eliminate even more fat from your diet, experiment with reducing the amount of oil or margarine called for in the recipes. Most of the recipes will fare admirably with less, even though we have already minimized the amounts used.

You can further reduce the quantity of oil used to prepare pan-fried or sautéed dishes by using a nonstick spray and/or a nonstick skillet. In addition, we suggest using a natural, nonstick spray instead of greasing the pan with oil when making

Lemonaid

Add a bit of dried lemon zest, lemon balm, lemon verbena, or lemon-scented pelargoniums to your favorite potpourri recipe for a fresh lemony fragrance.

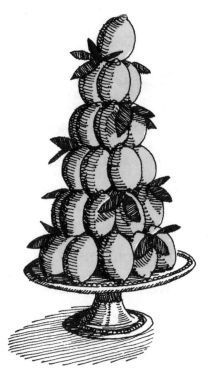

baked goods. (Natural, nonaerosol sprays of vegetable lecithin are available in most supermarkets and health food stores.)

Making Healthy Substitutions

There are a number of ingredient substitutions you can make to accommodate your own taste preferences and health needs. For example, we use eggs in a few of the recipes. But for those who prefer absolutely no animal-based products in their diets, a vegetarian egg substitute can be used in place of the eggs in most of the baked-goods recipes in this book. Here are more of our product preferences and the substitutions you may want to consider when reviewing the recipes:

Agar-agar—Available in bar, powder, and flake form, this tasteless sea vegetable is great as a jelling and thickening agent and is far superior to commercially available gelatins. We prefer the flake form in our recipes.

Arrowroot—We prefer arrowroot to processed cornstarch as a thickening agent. Arrowroot is a less-processed product. Of course, cornstarch may be substituted measure for measure for arrowroot if you don't mind the chemically treated and bleached product that is typically available in supermarkets.

Baking Powder—Look for a brand like Rumford that does not contain aluminum. Aluminum is toxic and should be avoided in your diet. Baking powders without aluminum are available in most supermarkets and health food stores.

Concentrated Fruit Sweetener—Natural concentrated fruit sweeteners are available in health food stores. These sweeteners may be made with one specific fruit such as apples or grapes, or may be a blend of different fruits. Because the blend contains several types of fruit, no one flavor stands out over another. Thus, we prefer the blend in our recipes as it doesn't overpower the lemon flavor. Concentrated fruit sweeteners are sweeter than malt or rice syrup, but not as sweet as honey.

Honey—While regarded by some as a health food, honey is primarily glucose and really not a whole lot better than white sugar. Honey does offer some trace vitamins and minerals that are not found in processed sugars. It is also a natural product, unlike chemically processed brown and white cane sugars.

Sucanat—This is a natural brown-sugar product prepared by dehydrating the juice of organically grown sugar cane. Unlike other processed cane sugars, Sucanat is a whole food. It's not as sweet as honey, but is sweeter than malt or date sugar. If you want a dish with date sugar to be sweeter, substitute Sucanat for the date sugar. We use Sucanat or date sugar instead of white sugar in most of our desserts. Sucanat adds color to a recipe that some may consider undesirable, but it also adds flavor and nutrition.

Soymilk—We use soymilk in many recipes as a substitute for dairy milk or cream. However, you can use organic nonfat cow's milk or nonfat goat's milk in one-to-one proportions in almost all of the recipes that call for soymilk. We do use Parmesan cheese, nonfat sour cream, and nonfat yogurt in some recipes. You can substitute silken tofu for the sour cream, tofu Parmesan for the regular Parmesan, and soy yogurt for the yogurt.

Shoyu and Tamari Sauce—The tastes of these sauces are similar. If a recipe calls for one, it's okay to use the other. As both shoyu (wheat-free soy sauce) and tamari (soy sauce with wheat) are high in salt, we suggest you use them in moderation.

Beans—One type of bean is easily substituted for another in almost every recipe that calls for beans. The recipe will look and taste different, but the results are sure to be tasty.

Lemon Vegetable Broth—Many of our recipes call for Lemon Vegetable Broth. The recipe for the broth is on page 86. As a substitute, chicken broth or vegetable bouillon can be used successfully in our recipes—but be careful to use low-salt

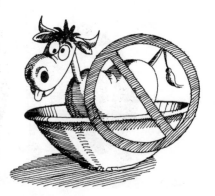

varieties. Many commercial broths and bouillons are very high in sodium. Of course, you can use your own favorite recipe for broth without adding lemon. We make a large pot of broth every week and keep some on hand as a base for soups and a flavoring for beans, grains, and main dishes.

Lemon Pepper and Other Lemony Substitutes—Lemon pepper (see page 227) can be substituted for fresh ground black pepper in any of the recipes. The reason it is not always suggested is that the taste of different lemon ingredients is lost when they are used on top of one another. Adding lemon juice, lemon zest, lemongrass, and lemon pepper to the same dish is redundant. It won't hurt anything—but it won't enhance anything either. You may prefer substituting lemon pepper for lemon zest or lemon mint for lemon juice. Experiment with the recipes and the lemon flavors. The nuance of the lemon flavor changes depending on the source.

Mock Lemon Butter—Mock Lemon Butter (actually made with soy margarine) is specified in small quantities in some of the recipes. You can also use it on toast, muffins, and vegetables, just as you would ordinary soy margarine. The recipe is on page 235. Put Mock Lemon Butter together as you're cooking and use it immediately, or whip it together ahead of time and let it sit to absorb more of the lemon flavor. Either way it's good, but when the margarine is allowed to "get acquainted" with the juice or zest, the lemon taste will be stronger. If you don't have time to make Mock Lemon Butter, use plain soy margarine in the recipes.

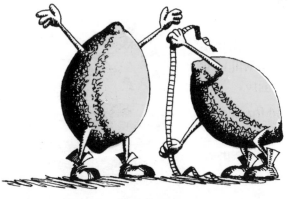

Salt—Almost none of our recipes contains added table salt. As we mentioned previously, the addition of lemon to your recipes enhances the taste of the foods while adding little or no sodium to the diet. If after adding all the lemon and herbs to a recipe you feel it still needs salt, first let the flavors blend for a few more minutes, then adjust the seasonings.

Don't be so quick to reach for the salt shaker. If you do choose to add salt, we recommend using only natural sea salt.

Measuring Your Lemons

The size of an average store-bought lemon is considered to be medium. Three or four of these lemons weigh one pound. You can sometimes find the larger Ponderosa lemons in the grocery store, but our recipes assume that you will use a medium lemon that yields the following:

1 medium lemon = almost ¼ cup of juice and
                   1 tablespoon of grated zest

3 medium lemons = about ½ cup of juice and
                  3 tablespoons of grated zest

6 medium lemons = just over 1 cup of juice and
                  6 tablespoons of grated zest

These are just averages. Lemons may be graded differently in different parts of the country. And a medium lemon from a backyard tree may yield a half cup of juice by itself. As a rule, a recipe calling for the juice of one lemon is asking for about a quarter cup. Feel free to adjust the amount you use to suit your taste.

The recipes in this book are meant to be guidelines to help you create your own masterpieces. As any good cook will tell you, there are no exact rules in cooking, and your taste and preference is just that—*your* taste and preference. Vary the amounts of juice and zest used in the recipes until you get the exact taste sensation that appeals to you. Experiment with different kinds and amounts of lemon-flavored and regular herbs. If you like the way a recipe sounds but don't particularly like one of the herbs or spices used, just go ahead and leave that herb or spice out.

How to Follow the Recipes

We suggest you read a recipe through several times before you start following the instructions. Get a feel for it and decide if there are substitutions you're going to make. Check that you have the key ingredients ready before you start mixing.

The serving amounts and preparation times provided in the recipes are averages. And if we say that a recipe will serve four, we mean four hearty eaters. You may get six servings if your family has smaller appetites.

Preparation times will vary depending on how you pace yourself. Cooking time will depend a great deal on your cookware and the characteristics of your oven or burners. Please do not interpret our times as hard-and-fast rules—you need to test your dish for doneness and adjust the times to the performance of your own kitchen.

There is only one ironclad rule in the kitchen. Experiment! Adjust the recipes in any way that makes sense to you. Of course, always use fresh lemons, herbs, and vegetables in your dishes if at all possible. There is simply no substitute for fresh.

Take a Chance

Every one of our recipes has a *Take a Chance* section. This section offers guidelines to help you in your own creative manipulations of the recipes. We suggest that you jot down the changes you make when you do create a masterpiece so that you can refresh your memory when you next crave that dish. There will be a next time, we promise.

No matter how you slice it, dice it, chop it, or zest it, the lemon is one of the most versatile foods in your kitchen. Lemons will always be there to brighten not only your culinary creations, but your life.

Chapter 3

Beverages With Lemon Juice—
A Drop of Liquid Gold

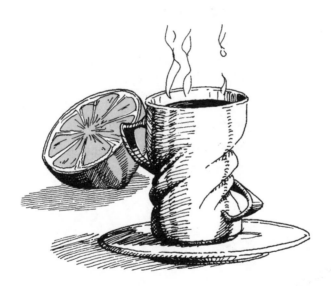

Lemon juice is by far the most refreshing and thirst-quenching liquid around. By itself, lemon juice may not be very appealing. But nothing in the world satisfies like a refreshing glass of lemonade on a hot summer day or a steaming cup of hot lemony tea during the long, cold winter. Use this precious liquid gold in the following recipes for a taste of sunshine on any day of the year.

Perfectly Refreshing Lemonade

Lemonade is so much more thirst-quenching than other drinks because of the abundance of citric acid in the lemons.

juice of 6 medium lemons

3 tablespoons concentrated fruit sweetener

4 cups cold water

ice cubes

4 mint sprigs

SERVES: 4   PREPARATION TIME: $1\frac{1}{4}$ HOURS

1 In a large pitcher, combine the lemon juice, concentrated fruit sweetener, and cold water. Stir until thoroughly mixed. More lemon juice can be added to taste.

2 Refrigerate the mixture for 1 hour, or until chilled.

3 Pour the lemonade into tall ice-filled glasses, garnish with the mint, and serve immediately.

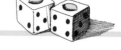

TAKE A CHANCE:

○ To give your lemonade even more flavor, don't discard the juiced lemon hulls. Instead, add them to the lemonade mixture in the pitcher. Strain the lemonade before serving.

○ Grate some lemon zest before juicing the lemons and add the zest to the lemonade.

○ Make Perfect Pink Lemonade by adding 1 tablespoon cherry or cranberry juice to each glass.

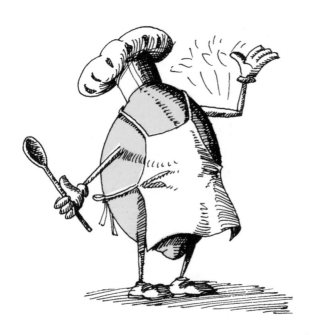

Lemonade Syrup

Lemonade has always been a summertime treat. With this syrup on hand, you can quickly mix up a glass of fresh-tasting lemonade at any time.

½ cup boiling water

¼ cup Sucanat

juice of 9 medium lemons

grated zest of 2 medium lemons

SERVES: 8   PREPARATION TIME: 20 MINUTES

1 Place the boiling water in a 16-ounce canning jar and add the Sucanat. Cover the jar and shake until combined.

2 Add the lemon juice and zest to the Sucanat syrup and shake until mixed. Cool to room temperature. Freeze the syrup in a plastic container (for up to 6 weeks) until needed.

3 To make lemonade by the glass, put ¼ cup of the syrup in a tall ice-filled glass. Add ¾ cup of cold water and stir.

4 To make lemonade by the pitcher, combine all of the syrup with 6 cups of cold water in a large pitcher. Mix well. Pour into ice-filled glasses.

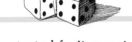

TAKE A CHANCE:

- Use ¼ cup date sugar, honey, or concentrated fruit sweetener instead of the Sucanat.

- Add more grated lemon zest to the syrup base.

- Mix the syrup base with sparkling mineral water, quinine water, or sparkling lemon-lime mineral water instead of plain water. Or try using one of these ingredients instead of plain water to make the ice cubes.

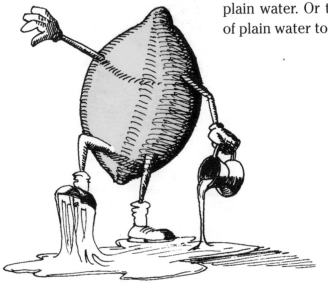

Lemon Cranberry Cooler

This tangy quencher is great on hot summer days. Mix up a batch and take it on a picnic.

ice cubes

2 cups cranberry juice

2 cups sparkling lemon-lime mineral water

4 lemon slices cut $\frac{1}{4}$-inch thick

4 mint sprigs

SERVES: 4   PREPARATION TIME: 5 MINUTES

1 Fill four tall glasses with equal amounts of the ice. Put ½ cup each of the cranberry juice and sparkling lemon-lime mineral water in each glass and mix well.

2 Float a lemon slice on top of each serving. Garnish with the mint and serve immediately.

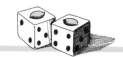

TAKE A CHANCE:

● Try freezing whole cranberries or quartered lemon slices in the ice cubes.

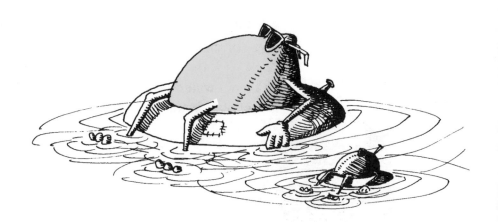

Half-and-Half Iced Tea

For those of you who like a real lemon kick with your iced tea, this version is a refreshing twist. With this tea, the taste of lemon doesn't quit.

1 cup Lemonade Syrup
(see page 35)

1 cup cold water

4 cups prepared herb or orange pekoe tea, cooled to room temperature

2 medium lemons, cut into wedges

ice cubes

4 mint sprigs

SERVES: 4   PREPARATION TIME: 10 MINUTES

1 Mix the Lemonade Syrup and cold water in a small pitcher and stir. Add the tea and stir well.

2 Add a wedge or two of the lemon to each of four tall ice-filled glasses. Pour the tea mixture into the glasses, garnish with the remaining lemon wedges and the mint, and serve immediately.

TAKE A CHANCE:

- Freeze lemon zest, cherries, or strawberries in the ice cubes.

- Omit the Lemonade Syrup and cold water and instead use 1 cup Perfectly Refreshing Lemonade (see page 34).

Lemonaid

A lemon slice added to a glass of water refreshes the mouth and cleanses the palate while eating.

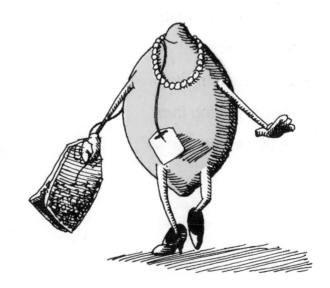

Citrus Slushies

Why give your kids a store-bought slushy that's full of artificial ingredients when this all-natural icy treat is so easy and economical to make at home?

juice of 2 medium lemons

1 cup orange juice

½ cup grapefruit juice

3 cups water

16 ice cubes

SERVES: 4 PREPARATION TIME: 10 MINUTES

1 Mix the juices and water together in a blender or food processor. Add the ice cubes and blend the mixture, in batches if necessary, until it is slushy.

2 Pour the mixture into paper cups or small glass dessert bowls and serve immediately.

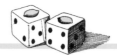

TAKE A CHANCE:

- Try adding a bit of grated citrus zest for some extra tang and visual interest.

- Add tiny pieces of citrus pulp to the blender.

- Try making the slushy with a small amount of Lemon Fruit Syrup (see page 244).

Lemonaid

Lemons have a high citric-acid content, making them more thirst-quenching than any other fruit.

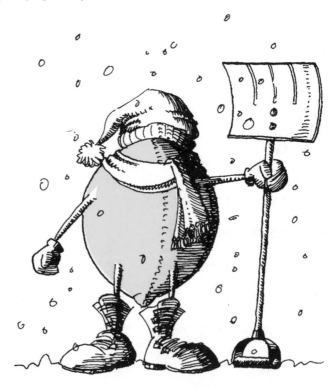

Old-Fashioned Lemon Barley Water

In days of yore, lemon barley water was a common folk cure for most indigestion and kidney problems. Today it is just a tasty way to get the benefits of lemons.

½ cup pearl barley

grated zest and juice of 2 medium lemons

10 cups cold water

2 teaspoons concentrated fruit sweetener

SERVES: 4   PREPARATION TIME: 1½ HOURS

1 Wash the barley under cold running water for 1 minute.

2 Put the barley and the lemon zest in a large pot with the 10 cups of water and bring to a boil. Reduce the heat to medium. Simmer uncovered, stirring occasionally so the barley does not scorch the pan, until half the liquid remains.

3 Strain the liquid into a pitcher or other serving container and discard the barley.

4 Add the lemon juice and concentrated fruit sweetener. Refrigerate until very cold and serve. The liquid may be poured into sterilized bottles and capped if you don't want to drink it right away.

TAKE A CHANCE:

- Sweeten with a bit of honey to taste.
- Garnish with sprigs of mint.

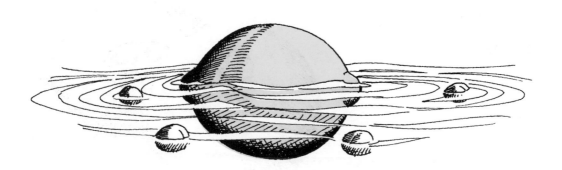

The Dynamic Citrus Duo

Who said that morning fruit juice has to be ordinary? This combination will send you on your way with a sunny spring in your step.

juice of 2 medium lemons

1⅔ cups orange juice

SERVES: 4   PREPARATION TIME: 5 MINUTES

1 Mix the juices and taste. Adjust sweetness by adding more orange juice, if desired.

2 Pour into tall glasses and serve immediately.

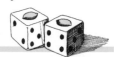

TAKE A CHANCE:

● Don't limit this Dynamic Duo to breakfast. Pour it over ice cubes, garnish it with mint or nasturtium leaves, and enjoy it any time of the day.

● Float some strawberry slices on top.

● Add ½ cup sparkling mineral water for a little fizz.

● Add some grated citrus zest for more appeal.

Lemonaid

Mound some of your excess lemons in a bowl or basket for use as a bright, sunny centerpiece.

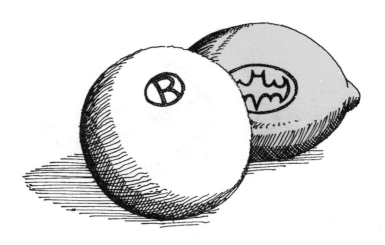

A Very Tart Virgin Mary

This drink is satisfying any time of any day, but we like it best with Sunday brunch.

juice of 1 medium lemon

4 cups tomato juice

1 teaspoon Worcestershire sauce

ice cubes

4 lemon slices cut $\frac{1}{4}$ -inch thick

4 celery stalks with leaves

SERVES: 4   PREPARATION TIME: 5 MINUTES

1 Combine the lemon juice, tomato juice, and Worcestershire sauce in a small pitcher and mix thoroughly.

2 Pour the Virgin Mary into tall ice-filled glasses. Garnish with the lemon slices and celery, and serve immediately.

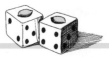

TAKE A CHANCE:

● Use a Moroccan Preserved Lemon (see page 246) for the juice.

● Add a few drops of hot sauce or stir in a bit of black pepper. Or add both!

● Use a slice of yellow or green bell pepper instead of the celery.

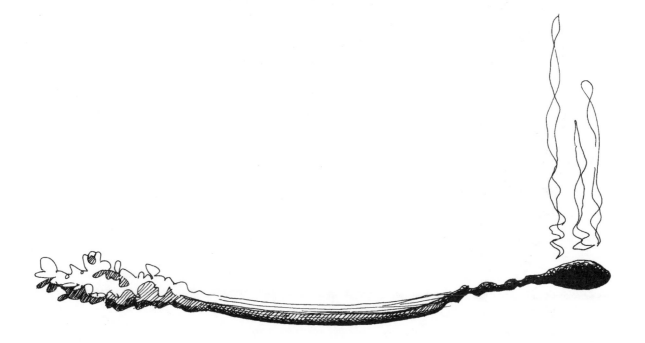

Basic Citrus Tea

othing is as satisfying on a cold morning as hot tea with lemon. You will have a hard time keeping your nose out of the steam coming off the cup.

½ teaspoon dried lemon and/or orange zest

4 teaspoons raspberry, chamomile, or herb tea of your choice

4 cups boiling water

4 lemon wedges

honey to taste (optional)

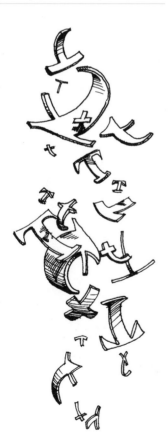

SERVES: 4   PREPARATION TIME: 10 MINUTES

1 Mix the dried zest with the loose tea and fill a large tea ball.

2 Pour the boiling water into a warm teapot. Add the tea ball and steep for 3 to 5 minutes. Remove the tea ball and pour the tea into a heated cup.

3 Squeeze out a lemon wedge into each cup of tea. The wedge can be added to the tea or discarded. Add the honey to taste, if desired, and serve hot.

TAKE A CHANCE:

- Add crushed cinnamon or a crumbled cinnamon stick to the tea ball, or sprinkle cinnamon in the cup.

- Add the zest of 1 grapefruit or 1 lime to the tea blend.

- Make a batch of hot tea and cool it for use as iced tea.

- If you don't mind caffeine, try loose orange pekoe tea instead of herb tea.

- Experiment with different herbs and spices—citrus zest blends with almost anything.

- Mix a large batch for future use. Just multiply the portions and keep the dry tea in a tightly sealed container.

Herbal Lemon Tea

his herbal mixture has a most heavenly lemon scent and is very soothing to frazzled nerves.

¼ cup dried lemon balm leaves

¼ cup dried lemon geranium leaves

¼ cup dried lemongrass

¼ cup dried lemon thyme leaves

¼ cup dried lemon verbena leaves

4 cups boiling water

SERVES: 4   PREPARATION TIME: 15 MINUTES

1 Mix all the herbs together and store in a tightly closed glass jar, out of the sunlight.

2 Use 2 teaspoons of the herbal mixture per cup of boiling water. Put the herbs in a teapot and pour the boiling water over the herbs. Cover the pot and steep for 5 to 10 minutes.

3 Strain the hot tea into a cup and serve immediately.

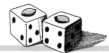

TAKE A CHANCE:

● Try this recipe with fresh herbs instead of the dried, using 1 tablespoon of the mixture for each 1 cup of tea.

● Add a small amount of dried lavender for a very exotic taste.

● Add a bit more of the herbs to the pot when brewing, then cool and serve as iced tea.

Lemonaid

Make an extra large batch of Herbal Lemon Tea. Use half of it for brewing and put the rest in a small dish for use as a lemony room freshener.

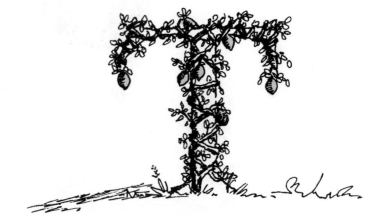

Citrus Honey Tea for a Crowd

Soothing and warming after skiing down the slopes or wrestling with a snowman. Invite the whole gang over!

12 cups water

2 cinnamon sticks

10 whole cloves

5 tea bags of your favorite herb or black tea

juice of 2 medium lemons

$\frac{1}{3}$ cup orange juice

3 tablespoons honey

1 medium lemon, thinly sliced

1 large orange, thinly sliced

SERVES: 16   PREPARATION TIME: 30 MINUTES

1 In a large pot, bring the water to a full boil. Lower the heat to a simmer and add the cinnamon, cloves, and tea bags. Steep for 5 minutes.

2 Strain the tea mixture into a large punch bowl and add the juices and honey, stirring until the honey dissolves.

3 Add half of the lemon and orange slices to the punch bowl. Garnish the cups with the remaining slices and serve.

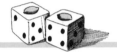

TAKE A CHANCE:

● Use 3 tablespoons date sugar or malt syrup instead of the honey.

● Try adding some whole allspice to the simmering water.

● Garnish each glass with a cinnamon stick.

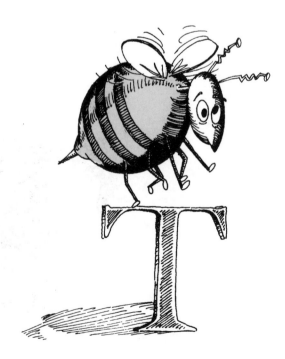

Wintertime Wassail

S oftly falling snow, a roaring fire, and a steaming cup of wassail—what more could anyone want? There doesn't even have to be a holiday in sight.

8 cinnamon sticks

2 tablespoons whole cloves

4 whole allspice

16 cups organic apple cider

juice of 8 medium lemons

$1\frac{1}{3}$ cups orange juice

$\frac{1}{4}$ cup Sucanat

$\frac{1}{2}$ medium lemon, cut into thin slices, then cut in half again

16 cinnamon sticks

SERVES: 16   PREPARATION TIME: 45 MINUTES

1 Wrap the 8 cinnamon sticks, cloves, and allspice together in a piece of cheesecloth and tie closed.

2 Put the cider and the wrapped spices in a large pot and simmer on low for 10 minutes, stirring occasionally.

3 Add the juices and Sucanat. Bring the mixture almost to a boil, then lower the heat and simmer for 20 minutes.

4 Ladle the wassail into warm mugs, garnish each with a lemon slice and cinnamon stick, and serve immediately.

TAKE A CHANCE:

- Use frozen lemon and orange juice instead of the fresh.
- Float whole lemon or orange slices studded with whole cloves and allspice on top of the punch.

Lemonaid

It takes approximately six lemons to make one cup of juice.

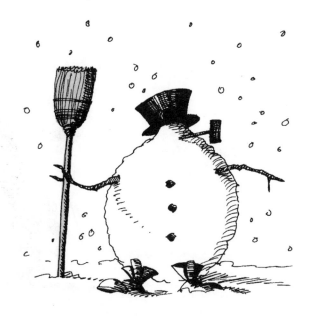

Wedding Punch

Don't wait for a wedding to make this punch. It will surely brighten up any occasion.

8 cups Perfectly Refreshing Lemonade (see page 34)

4 cups orange juice

4 cups pineapple juice

2 cups unfiltered organic apple juice

4 cups sparkling natural ginger ale

8 cups sparkling mineral water

Lemon Ice Ring (see page 50)

SERVES: 16   PREPARATION TIME: 10 MINUTES

1 Mix all the ingredients except the ice ring in a punch bowl. Adjust the amounts to taste.

2 Add the Lemon Ice Ring and serve.

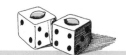

TAKE A CHANCE:

- Instead of the ice ring, use ice cubes made from plain water or sparkling mineral water and strawberries.

- Float lemon slices, orange slices, strawberries, or thin apple wedges in the punch.

- Use 1 cup puréed strawberries instead of the apple juice.

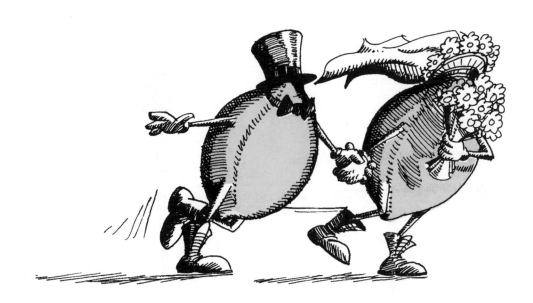

Honey of a Lemon Punch

Mix up this punch for your next big pool party—it's light and refreshing.

¼ cup water

¼ cup honey

juice of 6 medium lemons

1⅔ cups orange juice

¼ cup grapefruit juice

4 cups sparkling mineral water

24 ice cubes

SERVES: 8   PREPARATION TIME: 20 MINUTES

1 Heat the water to boiling and mix with the honey. This will help the honey dissolve faster. Set aside.

2 Combine all the remaining ingredients except the ice in a large bowl and mix well. Add the honey mixture and mix again. Let the punch stand for 10 minutes.

3 Stir well, add the ice cubes, and serve immediately.

TAKE A CHANCE:

● Float lemon or orange slices in the punch.

● Add sliced strawberries to the punch bowl.

● Freeze grated citrus zest or whole zest in the ice cubes.

● Use ice cubes made from sparkling mineral water, quinine water, or sparkling lemon-lime mineral water instead of plain water.

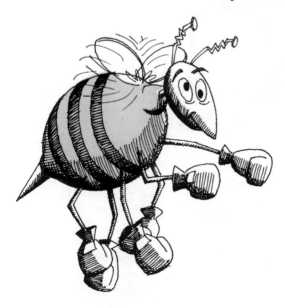

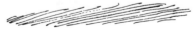

Spicy Hot Lemon Cranberry Punch

This is perfect for the tailgate party before the big game. It will help to keep the frost off your nose and your toes.

7 cups water

1 cup unfiltered organic apple juice

25 whole cloves

1 cinnamon stick, crushed with a rolling pin

juice of 3 medium lemons

1 cup cranberry juice

1 medium lemon, thinly sliced

SERVES: 8   PREPARATION TIME: 20 MINUTES

1 In a medium-sized saucepan, combine the water, the apple juice, 15 of the whole cloves, and the cinnamon stick. Bring to a boil and continue boiling for 5 minutes.

2 Strain the mixture into a punch bowl. Add the lemon juice and cranberry juice and stir.

3 Stud the lemon slices with the remaining whole cloves and float in the punch. Serve immediately while nice and hot.

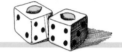

TAKE A CHANCE:

- Try using ¼ cup malt syrup instead of the apple juice.

- Add the zest of 1 or 2 lemons to the saucepan.

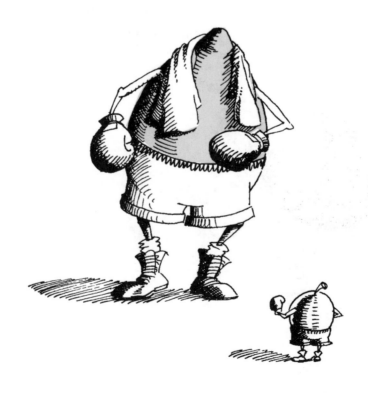

Citrus Sangria Olé

This alcohol-free sangria will be great fun at your next fiesta grande!

2 cups unfiltered organic apple juice

8 cups sparkling mineral water

juice of 8 medium lemons

$1\frac{1}{3}$ cups orange juice

2 medium lemons, sliced

2 large oranges, sliced

2 large limes, sliced

3 large peaches or nectarines, sliced

1 pint strawberries, hulled and sliced

15 cherries, pitted

30 ice cubes

SERVES: 16   PREPARATION TIME: 45 MINUTES

1 Place the apple juice and sparkling mineral water in a punch bowl and stir well.

2 Add all the remaining ingredients except the ice to the apple juice mixture and adjust for taste.

3 Refrigerate the sangria for 30 minutes.

4 Add the ice cubes to the bowl, stir, and serve immediately.

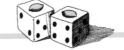

TAKE A CHANCE:

○ Add mint leaves to the punch.

○ Add apple wedges or grapes to the punch.

○ Freeze grated lemon and orange zest in the ice cubes.

○ Use sparkling mineral water for the ice cubes instead of plain water.

○ Use a Lemon Ice Ring (see page 50) instead of the plain ice cubes.

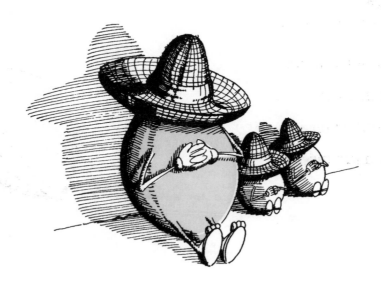

Lemon Ice Ring

A crowd pleaser for most any occasion, this colorful ice ring turns a simple punch into a lavish centerpiece.

4 medium lemons, thinly sliced

2 large oranges, thinly sliced

2 large limes, thinly sliced

12 cherries, pitted

cold water

YIELD: 1 LARGE RING   PREPARATION TIME: 4 HOURS

1 In a ring mold, arrange the citrus slices and cherries in an alternating pattern or a design of your choice. Pour just enough cold water into the mold to partially cover the fruit. Freeze until solid.

2 Remove the mold from the freezer and add more cold water until the mold is about ¾ full. Freeze until solid.

3 Unmold the ice ring by dipping quickly in warm water, then float the ring in a punch bowl filled with your favorite punch.

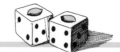

TAKE A CHANCE:

- Add mint leaves to the mold.
- Try using strawberries or blueberries instead of the cherries.
- Use sparkling mineral water instead of the plain water.
- Cut the fruit into smaller pieces and freeze it in ice cube trays instead of in a ring mold.

Lemonaid

Lemon-flavored herbs can be added to unsweetened fruit juices for a tart twist.

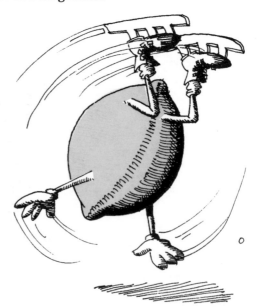

Chapter 4

Appetizers, Salads, and Sandwiches— Start With a Lemon Kick

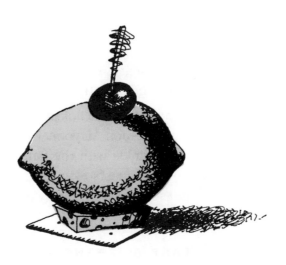

It's easy to jazz up the taste of appetizers, salads, and sandwiches with a few drops of lemon juice or a sprinkling of lemon zest. The bright taste of lemon heightens the flavor of all your recipes, and the refreshing fragrance will have your family and friends clamoring for more.

Baby Artichokes Dipped in Lemon Mayonnaise

emon Mayonnaise enhances the artichoke's subtle flavor. This recipe works just as well with bigger 'chokes, which can be a meal in themselves. Just increase the cooking time to allow for the size of the artichokes.

4 small artichokes

juice of $\frac{1}{2}$ medium lemon

4 teaspoons Lemon Mayonnaise (see page 237)

2 teaspoons chopped fresh parsley

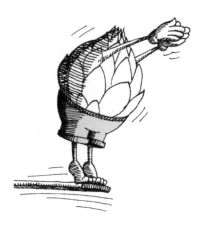

SERVES: 4   PREPARATION TIME: 45 MINUTES

1 Using a sharp knife, cut the top leaves off the artichokes about 1 inch down. Discard any small leaves at the base and trim the stems flush with the bottoms so the artichokes will stand upright. Using scissors, snip off all the thorn-like leaf ends. Brush the artichokes with the lemon juice to prevent discoloration.

2 Place the artichokes in a large pot containing enough boiling water to cover them and cook uncovered for 25 minutes, or until tender. The water should stay at a gentle boil. Drain the artichokes upside-down in a strainer until cool enough to handle.

3 When cool, slightly spread the artichoke leaves and remove the light green leaves in the center. Use a spoon to scrape out the tough spines at the center of the artichoke, then discard. Be careful not to scrape out the good green heart underneath the spines.

4 Arrange the artichokes on a serving plate. Place 1 teaspoon of the Lemon Mayonnaise in the center of each artichoke and sprinkle with the parsley. Serve immediately, instructing your guests to pull off a leaf, dip it in the mayonnaise, and scrape off the fleshy portion of the leaf with their teeth.

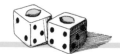

TAKE A CHANCE:

- Use chopped mint instead of the parsley.
- Drizzle olive oil on the leaves before serving.
- Add a few drops of Tabasco sauce to the Lemon Mayonnaise.
- Serve with a bowl of melted Mock Lemon Butter (see page 235) or Lemony Hollandaise Sauce (see page 230) instead of the mayonnaise.

Spicy Olives With Lemon Strips

S erve these olives as part of an appetizer plate. Or if you're looking for a new taste for an everyday salad, add a few of these treats for a little zing!

¼ cup extra virgin olive oil

juice of 2 medium lemons

zest of 1 medium lemon, slivered

2 large garlic cloves, minced

2 teaspoons chopped fresh rosemary

½ teaspoon crushed red pepper

2 whole black peppercorns

1 cup brine-cured black or green olives, drained and pitted

1 teaspoon minced fresh cilantro

SERVES: 4   PREPARATION TIME: 3¼ HOURS

1 Heat the oil in a small saucepan just until warm. Add the lemon juice, lemon zest, garlic, rosemary, red pepper, and peppercorns, and sauté for 2 minutes.

2 Place the olives in a small jar and cover with the marinade. Seal with a lid and refrigerate for 3 hours.

3 Remove the olives from the marinade and place them in a serving dish, sprinkle with the cilantro, and serve. If you manage to have any leftover olives, put them back in the jar and cover completely with olive oil. They can be kept in the refrigerator for several weeks.

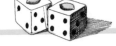

TAKE A CHANCE:

○ Use mushrooms instead of the olives.

○ Use parsley instead of the cilantro.

○ Use a few whole dried New Mexican red peppers instead of the crushed red pepper for a hotter olive.

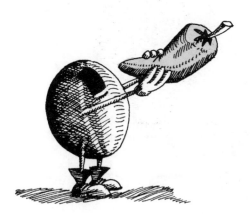

Lemony Marinated Mushrooms

By themselves or on a salad, these mushrooms truly have the spice of life—lemon!

1 pound mushrooms

juice of 1 medium lemon

2 large garlic cloves, minced

2 tablespoons light sesame or safflower oil

1 teaspoon dried thyme

SERVES: 4 PREPARATION TIME: 2¼ HOURS

1 Trim the stems of the mushrooms so that they are even with the caps. Leave the mushrooms whole if they are small, but cut them in halves or quarters if they are very large.

2 Place the lemon juice, garlic, oil, and thyme in a medium-sized bowl and stir well. Add the mushrooms and stir until they're thoroughly coated. Cover and refrigerate for 2 hours.

3 Stir well and serve.

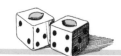

TAKE A CHANCE:

● Add 1 teaspoon grated lemon zest, 1 teaspoon crushed red pepper, and/or 1 tablespoon tomato paste to the marinade.

● Garnish with lemon balm.

Lemonaid

Lemon juice will remove the smell of garlic or onion from your hands.

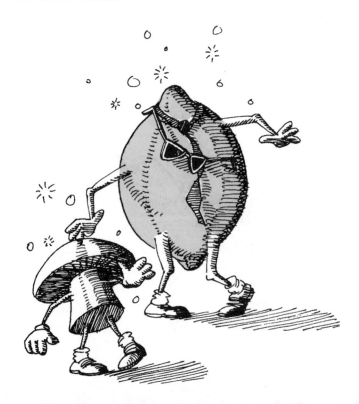

Hummus

A staple throughout the Middle East, hummus is great as a party dip. It also is a mainstay of vegetarian chefs everywhere—including those from Santa Cruz, California, where we discovered this recipe on a bulletin board in a surf shop.

grated zest and juice of 1 medium lemon

2 medium cucumbers, peeled, seeded, and chopped

2 large tomatoes, seeded and diced

½ teaspoon dried oregano

2 tablespoons safflower oil

3 large garlic cloves, minced

2 cups cooked chickpeas

1 cup tahini

4 drops hot sauce

¼ cup minced fresh cilantro

½ medium lemon, sliced

SERVES: 4   PREPARATION TIME: 20 MINUTES

1 Place the lemon zest, cucumber, tomato, and oregano in a small bowl and mix with 1 tablespoon of the lemon juice and 1 tablespoon of the oil. Set aside.

2 Place the remaining lemon juice and the garlic, chickpeas, tahini, and hot sauce in a blender or the bowl of a food processor and pulse until smooth. (Add more lemon juice or hot sauce if the mixture is too dry.)

3 Mound the chickpea mixture on a medium-sized serving plate and drizzle with the remaining oil. Arrange the cucumber-tomato salad around the hummus. Garnish with the cilantro and lemon slices, and serve with whole grain crackers, pita bread, or raw vegetables.

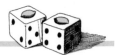

TAKE A CHANCE:

- Add more hot sauce for greater zing.
- Chop pitted Greek or Italian black olives and add to the cucumber salad.
- Add 1 teaspoon cumin to the chickpeas.
- Add minced parsley to the chickpeas.
- Use the drained cooking liquid from the chickpeas to thin the mixture.
- For a low-fat hummus, reduce the tahini to ¼ cup and eliminate the oil.
- Use sprouted chickpeas for easier digestion.

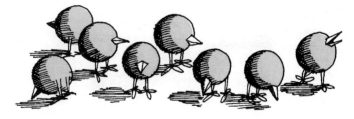

Spicy Crushed Chickpeas

This chunky mixture makes a delicious dip for raw vegetables and a wonderful appetizer with crackers or toasted pita. For a real treat, use it in Crunchy Lemon Sandwiches (see page 82) instead of tofu.

2 cups cooked chickpeas

juice of 1 medium lemon

2 large garlic cloves, finely minced

1 teaspoon dried marjoram

1 tablespoon light sesame or safflower oil

$\frac{1}{4}$ teaspoon freshly ground black pepper

$\frac{1}{2}$ cup finely minced fresh parsley

SERVES: 4   PREPARATION TIME: 45 MINUTES

1 In a small serving bowl, mash the chickpeas lightly with a fork. They should still be chunky.

2 Add all the remaining ingredients except the parsley to the chickpeas and mix well. Cover and chill for 30 minutes.

3 Mix the spread, adding a few drops of oil if it seems too thick. Garnish with the parsley and serve immediately with whole wheat crackers or raw vegetables.

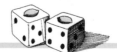

TAKE A CHANCE:

- Add a finely diced small red or green jalapeño pepper.
- Add a few drops of Tabasco sauce or some cayenne pepper.
- Use cilantro instead of the parsley.
- Add 2 tablespoons chopped onion.
- Add ¼ teaspoon ground cumin.

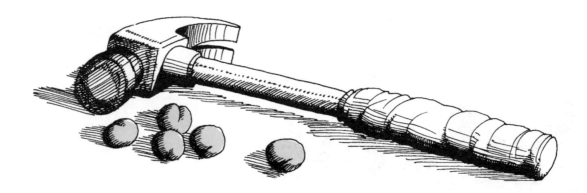

Zesty Lemon Dip

Getting tired of the same old dips? Try this to eliminate the chip-and-dip doldrums.

2 cups nonfat cottage cheese or nonfat yogurt

grated zest of 1 medium lemon

juice of $\frac{1}{2}$ medium lemon

2 scallions, finely minced

$\frac{1}{4}$ teaspoon hot sauce

$\frac{1}{4}$ teaspoon freshly ground black pepper

2 tablespoons finely chopped fresh parsley

SERVES: 4   PREPARATION TIME: 45 MINUTES

1 Place the cottage cheese or yogurt in a medium-sized bowl and stir vigorously until creamy. Add all the remaining ingredients except the parsley and mix well.

2 Cover the mixture and refrigerate for at least 30 minutes.

3 Stir well and garnish with the parsley. Serve with raw vegetables or whole grain crackers.

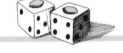

TAKE A CHANCE:

Try adding 2 to 3 tablespoons minced cucumber or green bell pepper.

Add fresh or dried thyme.

Garnish with chili powder or cayenne pepper.

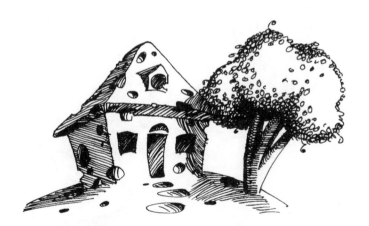

Lemonaid

Lemons don't sweeten after being picked.

Zesty Guacamole

Y ou can't live in the Phoenix area, as we do, and not serve guacamole often. A touch of lemon in your guacamole not only gives it a wonderful tang, but it also keeps it from turning brown. Serve with organic tortilla chips or fresh vegetables.

4 ripe medium avocados, peeled and pitted

juice of 1 medium lemon

3 large garlic cloves, finely minced

$\frac{1}{2}$ cup finely minced onion

2 large tomatoes, seeded and finely chopped

6 drops hot sauce

$\frac{1}{8}$ teaspoon freshly ground black pepper

2 tablespoons finely chopped fresh parsley

SERVES: 4   PREPARATION TIME: 1$\frac{1}{2}$ HOURS

1 In a small bowl, mash the avocados with a fork or a large spoon until almost smooth.

2 Add all the remaining ingredients except the parsley to the avocados and stir vigorously. If the mixture seems too dry, add another teaspoon of lemon juice. Cover and refrigerate for at least 1 hour so the flavors can blend.

3 Stir lightly, garnish with the parsley, and serve with whole grain chips or raw vegetables.

TAKE A CHANCE:

● Add 2 to 3 finely chopped red or green jalapeño peppers.

● Omit the tomatoes.

● Use cilantro instead of the parsley.

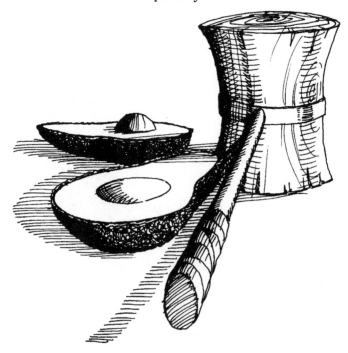

*F*resh Lemony Salsa

This salsa is quick and easy to make, so we use it on almost everything. It will keep 2 to 3 days in the refrigerator but is best when served fresh.

4 large tomatoes, seeded and coarsely chopped

2 large garlic cloves, minced

$\frac{1}{4}$ cup finely chopped onion

2 large red or green jalapeño peppers, seeded and finely chopped

$\frac{1}{4}$ cup finely minced fresh cilantro

juice of 1 medium lemon

SERVES: 4   PREPARATION TIME: 1$\frac{1}{2}$ HOURS

1 Place all the ingredients in a medium-sized glass bowl or jar and stir well. Cover and refrigerate for 1 hour.

2 Stir well and serve as a dip with organic tortilla chips, or use as a condiment or sauce for a main dish or vegetable.

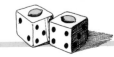

TAKE A CHANCE:

Add more jalapeños for a spicier salsa.

Add 1 teaspoon lemon zest for color and tang.

Use as a low-calorie topping for baked potatoes.

Lemonaid

A medium-sized lemon weighs about a quarter of a pound.

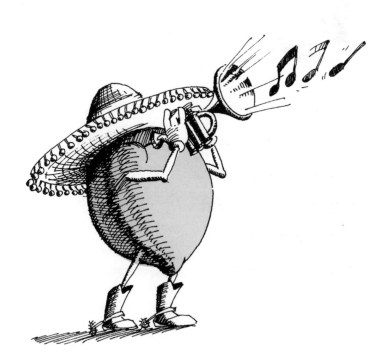

Zesty Eggplant Dip

Combining roasted eggplant with tahini (sesame seed paste), this wonderful dip is a lemony version of Baba Ghanoush. Make plenty, because it'll go fast!

1 large eggplant

juice of 1 medium lemon

3 large garlic cloves, chopped

1 tablespoon minced fresh cilantro

$\frac{1}{2}$ cup tahini

$\frac{1}{2}$ teaspoon ground cumin

SERVES: 4   PREPARATION TIME: 2$\frac{1}{2}$ HOURS

1 Using a fork, pierce the eggplant several times. Bake in a 350°F oven for 1 hour, or until the eggplant is soft, turning the eggplant several times during the baking process.

2 Allow the eggplant to cool, then peel, chop, and mash it in a bowl. Add the lemon juice, garlic, cilantro, tahini, and cumin, and mix well. Cover and chill for 1 hour.

3 Mix the salad well once again and serve as a spread with toasted pita bread or crackers, or use as a dip with raw vegetables.

TAKE A CHANCE:

• For a smoky flavor, roast the eggplant on a barbecue grill or over an open flame.

• Add 1 tablespoon minced onion.

• Add 1 teaspoon grated lemon zest.

• Add 1 minced red or green jalapeño pepper.

Lemonaid

When using lemon zest in a recipe, be sure not to include any of the white part (pith) or the dish will have a bitter taste.

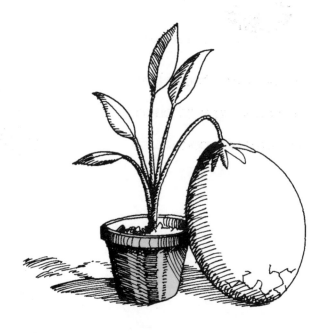

Jalapeño Pepper Jelly

This colorful jelly combines two Southwestern favorites—jalapeños and lemon. A festive-looking treat, it's wonderful when spread over tofu cheese and crackers. It does contain a lot of sugar, but a little goes a long way. It will keep for months in the refrigerator.

1 large green bell pepper, seeded and coarsely chopped

3 large green jalapeño peppers, seeded and coarsely chopped

$\frac{1}{2}$ cup apple cider vinegar

$1\frac{1}{2}$ cups date sugar

juice of 2 medium lemons

6 tablespoons liquid pectin

Lemonaid

Diluted lemon juice can be used as an astringent to help combat oily skin.

SERVES: 8   PREPARATION TIME: $3\frac{1}{4}$ HOURS

1 Place the bell and jalapeño peppers and the vinegar in a blender or the bowl of a food processor and blend until smooth.

2 Pour the mixture into a medium-sized saucepan. Add the date sugar and stir the mixture over medium heat until the sugar has dissolved, 2 to 3 minutes.

3 Add the lemon juice and bring the mixture to a boil for 5 minutes, stirring constantly.

4 Remove the saucepan from the heat and add the pectin, blending well. Pour the mixture into sterilized jars and refrigerate for 3 hours, or until set.

TAKE A CHANCE:

- Make the jelly hotter by leaving the seeds in the jalapeños.
- Make Red Pepper Jelly with red bell peppers and red jalapeños.
- Spread the jelly over tofu or Unmeatloaf With Lemon Sauce (see page 129) before grilling.

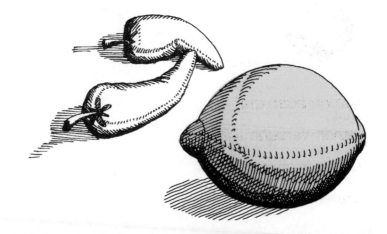

A Slice of Sunshine Salad

This tangy citrus salad will add gusto to any meal.

1 medium lemon, peeled, sectioned, and cut into pieces

2 medium grapefruits, peeled, sectioned, and cut into pieces

4 large oranges, peeled, sectioned, and cut into pieces

1 to 2 tablespoons orange juice to taste (optional)

mint leaves

SERVES: 4   PREPARATION TIME: 1½ HOURS

1 Combine the fruit in a large bowl.

2 Cover the fruit and refrigerate for 1 hour. If after chilling the fruit seems too tart, toss in the orange juice to sweeten the mixture.

3 Arrange the fruit on a medium-sized serving plate, garnish with the mint, and serve immediately.

TAKE A CHANCE:

- Add a few strawberries or tangerine sections for color.
- Add apple pieces for sweetness and crunch.

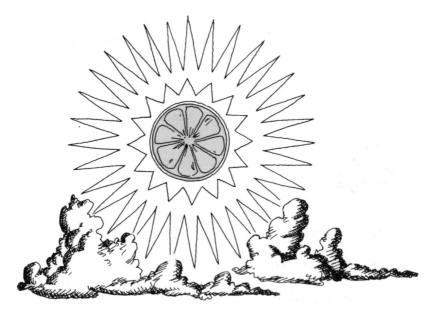

Lemonaid

Lemon balm and lemon verbena will add a fresh taste to fruit salads.

Lemon Antipasto

Translated literally, antipasto means "before the meal" and is intended to stimulate the appetite and make you eager for the next course. What better way to accomplish that than with an elegant combination of fresh vegetables enhanced by a lemony dressing?

Dressing

juice of 2 medium lemons

2 large garlic cloves, crushed

4 tablespoons extra virgin olive oil

2 tablespoons chopped fresh oregano, or
1 tablespoon dried

$\frac{1}{4}$ teaspoon freshly ground black pepper

Salad

1 head romaine lettuce, torn into pieces

1 medium onion, sliced

2 medium cucumbers, peeled and cut into spears

2 large tomatoes, cut into wedges

8 ounces asparagus, steamed and cooled to room temperature

1 medium red bell pepper, seeded and sliced

4 scallions, trimmed but left whole

6 ounces low-fat mozzarella cheese, sliced (optional)

12 brine-cured black olives (optional)

SERVES: 6 PREPARATION TIME: 20 MINUTES

1 Make the dressing by combining the lemon juice, garlic, oil, oregano, and black pepper in a small bowl. Allow the dressing to stand for 10 minutes.

2 Cover a large serving platter with the lettuce and arrange the vegetables in concentric circles on top. Roll the cheese slices and add them, along with the olives, to the arrangement, if desired.

3 Mix the dressing once again and pour it over the salad. Serve immediately.

TAKE A CHANCE:

- Sprinkle the antipasto with freshly grated Parmesan or Romano cheese.

- Garnish with wedges of hard-boiled egg.

- Add sliced mushrooms or carrots to the salad.

- Add fresh basil instead of the oregano to the dressing.

- For some spice, add 1 teaspoon crushed red pepper to the dressing.

- Add 1 teaspoon lemon zest to the dressing.

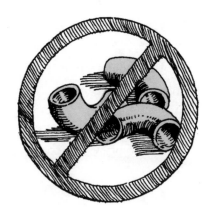

Greek Salad With a Lemon Tang

This salad doesn't get mixed in a bowl; instead, all the goodies are layered over the lettuce and then the lemon juice and oil are drizzled on top. While this recipe gives you a choice of lettuce, in Greece we were never served anything but the freshest, tastiest iceberg lettuce.

4 cups shredded lettuce (romaine, bibb, iceberg, or your choice)

6 red radishes, sliced

1 large green bell pepper, seeded and cut into $\frac{1}{2}$-inch strips

1 large tomato, cut into wedges

$\frac{1}{2}$ large cucumber, peeled and thinly sliced

4 onion slices, broken into rings

2 teaspoons chopped fresh oregano, or 1 teaspoon dried

4 slices ($\frac{1}{4}$-inch each) feta cheese

juice of 2 medium lemons

1 tablespoon extra virgin olive oil

$\frac{1}{4}$ cup Greek olives, or any other type of black olive, pitted

SERVES: 4　PREPARATION TIME: 25 MINUTES

1 Arrange the lettuce on four individual salad plates. Divide the radishes, green pepper, tomato, cucumber, and onion rings among the plates and arrange on top of the lettuce.

2 Sprinkle the oregano over the vegetables and top the salad with the feta cheese.

3 Mix the lemon juice and oil together in a small bowl and drizzle over each salad. *Do not toss!*

4 Garnish each dish with Greek olives and serve immediately.

TAKE A CHANCE:

○ The taste of this salad will change depending on the type of olive oil and the brand of feta cheese used. Experiment!

○ Crumble the feta cheese instead of slicing it.

○ Instead of mixing the lemon juice and oil together before adding them to the salad, just squeeze out the lemon over the salad and drizzle the oil on top. Each bite will taste a little different.

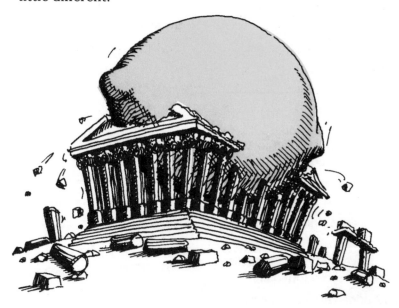

Romaine With Olive Oil and Lemon

The best part of this salad is eating the stuff left in the bottom of the bowl at the end of the meal when no one is looking. You have to use your fingers, of course!

juice of 1 medium lemon

1 large garlic clove, minced

2 tablespoons extra virgin olive oil

1 small tomato, seeded and diced

1 small green bell pepper, seeded and diced

1 medium head romaine lettuce, torn into bite-sized pieces

SERVES: 4 PREPARATION TIME: 20 MINUTES

1 Mix the lemon juice, garlic, and oil in a large bowl and let stand for 15 minutes.

2 Add all the remaining ingredients to the bowl, toss thoroughly, and serve.

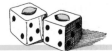

TAKE A CHANCE:

● Add 1 finely chopped shallot.

● Use red leaf lettuce.

● Add Lemon Garlic Croutons (see page 225).

● Top with 2 teaspoons freshly grated Romano cheese.

Lemonaid

Add more lemon juice to a recipe and you can decrease the oil needed. Add oil to a salad by using a spray bottle to spritz it on the greens.

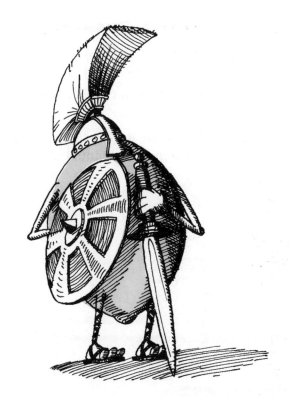

The Perfect Caesar Salad

Adjust the amounts of lemon and garlic in this salad to make it perfect for your taste.

juice of 1 medium lemon

2 large garlic cloves, crushed

2 tablespoons extra virgin olive oil

¼ teaspoon dry mustard

½ teaspoon Worcestershire sauce

¼ teaspoon freshly ground black pepper

1 large egg (optional)

1 large head romaine lettuce, torn into bite-sized pieces

2 tablespoons freshly grated Parmesan cheese

Lemon Garlic Croutons (see page 225)

Serves: 4 Preparation Time: 20 minutes

1 Combine the lemon juice, garlic, and oil in a large salad bowl—preferably a wooden one. Mix well and let stand for 15 minutes.

2 Add the dry mustard, Worcestershire sauce, and pepper to the bowl and mix well. Add the egg, if desired, and stir again, coating the sides of the bowl with the mixture.

3 Add the lettuce to the bowl and toss until the leaves are well coated. Sprinkle the cheese over the salad and toss.

4 Garnish with the croutons and serve immediately.

Note From a Healthy Lemon:

To make a cholesterol-free salad, replace the egg with an egg substitute, or eliminate the egg completely.

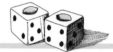

Take a Chance:

- If you would like a little less garlic, split a clove in half, rub the bowl with the cut sides, and then discard the clove.

- Use Romano cheese instead of the Parmesan for a sharper taste.

- Leave the lettuce leaves whole. Place them in a decorative pattern on individual plates and top with the dressing.

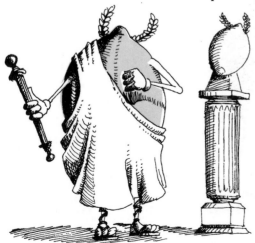

Wilted Citrus Spinach Salad

Take advantage of all that lovely fresh spinach now available almost all year long. Lemon and spinach are a great combination.

Dressing

3 tablespoons safflower oil

$\frac{1}{4}$ cup finely chopped onion

juice of $\frac{1}{2}$ medium lemon

Salad

1 pound fresh spinach leaves, torn into bite-size pieces

2 large oranges, peeled, sectioned, and cut into pieces

1 large hard-boiled egg, coarsely chopped

$\frac{1}{4}$ cup chopped walnuts

SERVES: 4 PREPARATION TIME: 25 MINUTES

1 To make the dressing, heat the oil in a small saucepan and sauté the onion until transparent, about 5 minutes. Remove the pan from the heat and stir in the lemon juice. Set aside.

2 To make the salad, place the spinach leaves in a large bowl along with the oranges. Add the warm dressing and mix well.

3 Garnish the salad with the egg and nuts, and serve immediately.

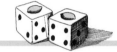

TAKE A CHANCE:

- Try adding slivered lemon and orange zest to the salad.
- Add a few pieces of sectioned lemon slices.
- Add diced red or yellow bell pepper or sliced mushrooms.
- Use sunflower seeds or pecans instead of the walnuts.
- Use Lemon Garlic Croutons (see page 225) instead of the walnuts.

Lemonaid

Whole lemons and lemon juice will lose some nutritional value when frozen.

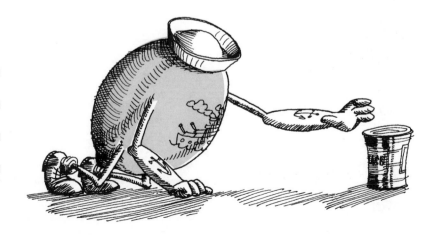

Daikon Radish Salad With a Lemon Twist

A white radish, the daikon picks up the flavor of the lemon and oil. If you can't find it at the grocery store, check out your local Asian market.

1½ cups grated daikon radish

10 red radishes, shredded

2 medium carrots, peeled and grated

3 tablespoons finely minced fresh cilantro

grated zest and juice of ½ medium lemon

2 teaspoons olive oil

¼ teaspoon Sucanat

¼ teaspoon freshly ground black pepper

SERVES: 4   PREPARATION TIME: 45 MINUTES

1 Drain the excess liquid from the grated daikon radish. Place the radish in a medium-sized bowl with the red radish and carrot, and mix. Set aside.

2 Mix all the remaining ingredients in a small bowl and pour over the vegetables. Adjust the seasonings, if necessary, then cover and refrigerate for 30 minutes.

3 Mix well and serve.

TAKE A CHANCE:

- Add 1 cup shredded green cabbage or Chinese (napa) cabbage, adjusting the other ingredients accordingly.

- Add ½ cup coarsely chopped celery.

- Reduce the olive oil and add ½ teaspoon sesame oil or hot chili pepper oil.

- Add ½ teaspoon cayenne pepper.

Lemonaid

Add more fresh zest to your cooking for a more intense lemon flavor.

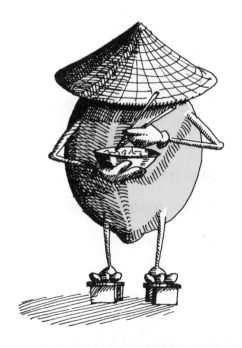

Party-Colored Lemon Cole Slaw

*T*his slaw is a feast for the eyes as well as the palate.

Dressing

grated zest and juice of 1 medium lemon

2 large garlic cloves, finely minced

$\frac{1}{4}$ cup Almost Sour Cream (see page 234)

$\frac{1}{4}$ cup silken tofu, mashed

1 teaspoon raspberry vinegar

1 teaspoon caraway seeds

$\frac{1}{4}$ teaspoon freshly ground black pepper

Salad

2 cups thinly sliced cabbage

1 cup thinly sliced red cabbage

1 medium red bell pepper, seeded and cut into $\frac{1}{4}$-inch strips

1 large carrot, peeled and grated

3 tablespoons minced fresh parsley

$\frac{1}{2}$ medium lemon, thinly sliced

SERVES: 4   PREPARATION TIME: 30 MINUTES

1 Make the dressing by combining the lemon zest, lemon juice, garlic, Almost Sour Cream, mashed tofu, vinegar, caraway seeds, and black pepper in a small bowl. Set aside.

2 Place the cabbage, red pepper, and carrot in a large bowl. Add the dressing and toss to mix.

3 Garnish the salad with the parsley and lemon slices, and serve.

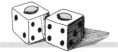

TAKE A CHANCE:

○ Use Lemon Mayonnaise (see page 237) instead of the Almost Sour Cream.

○ Add 1 to 2 diced fresh hot peppers to the salad or a few drops of hot sauce to the dressing, or both.

○ Add yellow or orange bell peppers, or try one of each.

○ Add the grated zest of 1 orange.

○ Garnish with toasted sesame seeds.

○ Add raisins that have been plumped in hot water.

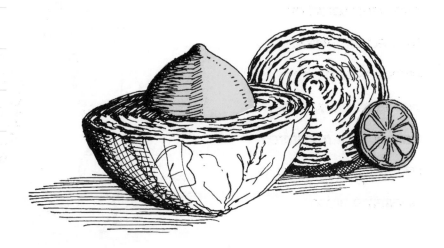

Grated Carrot Salad With Zesty Lemon

This is one salad that can be put together fast. And it's a refreshing change from lettuce-based affairs.

2 large carrots, peeled and grated

3 tablespoons finely chopped onion

1 teaspoon light sesame or safflower oil

3 tablespoons lemon juice

$\frac{1}{4}$ teaspoon freshly ground black pepper

SERVES: 4   PREPARATION TIME: 20 MINUTES

1 Place all the ingredients together in a bowl and stir.

2 Serve immediately, or cover and refrigerate for up to 1 day.

TAKE A CHANCE:

Add ½ teaspoon grated lemon zest.

Use 1 finely chopped shallot instead of the onion.

Lemonaid

Equal parts of lemon juice and salad oil rubbed into wood removes scratches. Try it first on a hidden part of your furniture, as it may discolor or dry some woods.

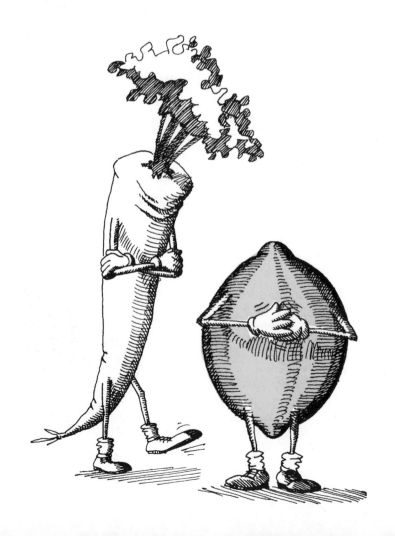

Broccoli Salad With Lemon and Garlic

A logical explanation has never been given, but Michelle insists that this salad must be made on a flat plate. Whatever type of dish you use, though, this garlicky salad is sure to be a hit.

juice of 6 medium lemons

8 large garlic cloves, finely minced

1 pound broccoli, trimmed and cut into 3-inch pieces and florets

SERVES: 4   PREPARATION TIME: $3\frac{1}{2}$ HOURS

1 Combine the lemon juice and garlic in a small bowl and set aside for 15 minutes.

2 Place the broccoli stems in a steamer for 2 minutes. Add the broccoli florets and steam for an additional 2 to 3 minutes. The broccoli should still be very crisp when removed from the steamer.

3 Arrange the steamed broccoli on a *flat* plate or dish and pour the marinade over the top. Cover and refrigerate for at least 3 hours, turning occasionally so that the broccoli marinates evenly.

4 Mix well and serve immediately.

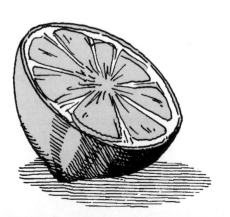

TAKE A CHANCE:

- Sprinkle with crushed red pepper before serving.

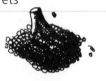

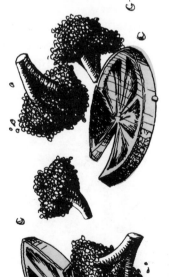

Lemon Tree Very Healthy Cookbook

Tomato and Green Pepper Salad With Moroccan Preserved Lemon

The Moroccan-style lemon gives this salad a wonderful taste that will have everyone clamoring for more.

Dressing

juice of 1 medium lemon

2 large garlic cloves, crushed

2 teaspoons extra virgin olive oil

2 tablespoons finely chopped fresh cilantro

$\frac{1}{4}$ teaspoon freshly ground black pepper

Salad

3 large tomatoes, seeded and diced

2 medium green bell peppers, seeded and diced

$\frac{1}{4}$ cup coarsely chopped onion

$\frac{1}{4}$ Moroccan Preserved Lemon (see page 246)

SERVES: 4 PREPARATION TIME: 45 MINUTES

1 Make the dressing by whisking together the lemon juice, garlic, oil, cilantro, and black pepper in a small bowl. Set aside.

2 Place the tomato, green pepper, and onion in a large bowl. Add the dressing and toss to mix.

3 Rinse the preserved lemon in cold water and remove the pulp. Cut the zest into tiny cubes and add to the salad. Cover and refrigerate for about 30 minutes so the flavors can blend.

4 Mix the salad well and serve immediately.

TAKE A CHANCE:

- If your batch of preserved lemons isn't ready yet, use the zest of 1 lemon instead.

- Give your peppers a smoky flavor by preparing them Moroccan-style. Grill them over a gas flame or bake them for 20 minutes until the skins are black and blistered. Remove the skins with a knife and dice the peppers.

- Add a coarsely chopped cucumber.

- Add a diced fresh hot pepper.

- Use parsley instead of the cilantro.

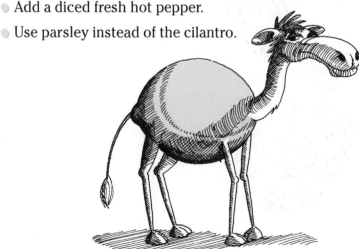

Lemon-Flecked Cucumber Salad

Fresh, crunchy cucumbers are always a healthy treat, but they're especially good when picked from your own garden. A little lemon dresses them up nicely.

Dressing

grated zest and juice of 1 medium lemon

1 teaspoon safflower oil

1 teaspoon balsamic vinegar

½ teaspoon chopped fresh oregano

Salad

2 medium cucumbers, peeled and thinly sliced

1 scallion, sliced

1 large garlic clove, finely chopped

SERVES: 4   PREPARATION TIME: 1¼ HOURS

1 Make the dressing by combining half of the lemon zest, all of the lemon juice, and the oil, vinegar, and oregano in a small bowl. Set aside.

2 Place the cucumber, scallion, and garlic in a medium-sized bowl. Add the dressing and toss to mix. Cover and refrigerate for at least 1 hour.

3 Toss the salad once again, garnish with the remaining lemon zest, and serve immediately.

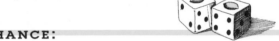

TAKE A CHANCE:

- Use dill instead of the oregano.
- Add 6 quartered cherry tomatoes.
- Use ½ cup sliced red, white, or yellow onion instead of the scallion.

Lemonaid

When filling your ice cube trays, add some lemon zest. The ice cubes look interesting and add a fresh flavor to any beverage as they melt.

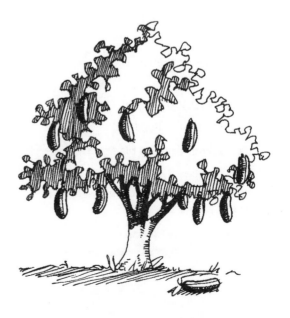

Fiesta Bean Salad

Double this nutritious, easy-to-make salad and take it to your next potluck supper.

Dressing

juice of 2 medium lemons

2 large garlic cloves, finely chopped

2 teaspoons light sesame or safflower oil

3 tablespoons finely minced fresh cilantro

$\frac{1}{4}$ teaspoon freshly ground black pepper

Salad

1 large red bell pepper, seeded and diced

1 large green bell pepper, seeded and diced

1 large red or green jalapeño pepper, seeded and diced

1 large tomato, seeded and diced

1 cup cooked corn

3 scallions, thinly sliced

1 cup cooked, drained black beans

1 cup cooked, drained Great Northern beans

SERVES: 4   PREPARATION TIME: 45 MINUTES

1 Make the dressing by combining the lemon juice, garlic, oil, cilantro, and black pepper in a small bowl. Set aside.

2 Place all the remaining ingredients in a large bowl. Add the dressing and toss to mix. Cover and let stand at room temperature for about 30 minutes.

3 Toss the salad once again and serve.

TAKE A CHANCE:

- Serve in a lettuce leaf or over chopped greens.
- Use a red onion instead of the scallions.
- Use yellow or orange bell peppers instead of the red or green ones.
- Add 1 tablespoon grated lemon zest to the dressing.
- Try parsley instead of the cilantro.
- Try pinto beans or rice instead of the Great Northern beans.

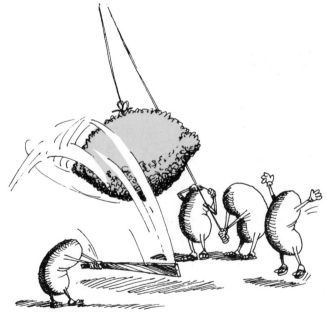

Lemony Lentil Salad

This wonderful salad is not only easy to make, it's also good for the lemon lover in you.

2 cups dried lentils, sorted and rinsed

juice of 3 medium lemons

$\frac{1}{4}$ teaspoon freshly ground black pepper

1 teaspoon extra virgin olive oil

3 medium garlic cloves, minced

2 scallions, coarsely chopped

1 teaspoon ground cumin

2 teaspoons extra virgin olive oil (optional)

SERVES: 4   PREPARATION TIME: 1 HOUR

1 Place the lentils in a medium-sized saucepan with enough water to cover. Bring to a boil, then simmer uncovered for 20 minutes, or until the lentils are tender. Drain and cool to room temperature.

2 Place the lentils in a medium-sized serving bowl and add the lemon juice and pepper. Mix well.

3 Heat the teaspoon of oil in a small saucepan and sauté the garlic, scallion, and cumin for 1 minute. Add the garlic mixture to the lentils and mix well. Cover and let stand at room temperature for 30 minutes.

4 Stir the mixture well, and serve. For a moister salad, drizzle the 2 teaspoons of olive oil over the lentils just before serving.

TAKE A CHANCE:

- Add 2 teaspoons chopped fresh parsley.
- Add a juiced lemon hull to the simmering lentils and remove it before serving.
- Use cayenne pepper instead of the cumin.
- Sprinkle with a chopped hard-boiled egg.

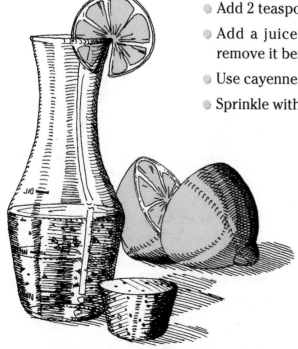

Sunny Rice Salad

D otted with splashes of bright zest, this colorful salad will help satisfy your lemon craving—at least for an hour or two.

Dressing

grated zest and juice of 1 medium lemon

1 large garlic clove, finely minced

2 teaspoons light sesame oil

$\frac{1}{2}$ teaspoon Dijon mustard

1 tablespoon rice vinegar

$\frac{1}{4}$ teaspoon freshly ground black pepper

Salad

3 cups cooked brown basmati rice, at room temperature

1 cup green peas

$\frac{1}{2}$ pound green beans, trimmed and blanched until just tender

$\frac{1}{4}$ cup coarsely chopped fresh mint

SERVES: 4   PREPARATION TIME: 2$\frac{1}{2}$ HOURS

1 Make the dressing by combining the lemon zest, lemon juice, garlic, oil, mustard, vinegar, and pepper in a small bowl. Mix thoroughly and set aside.

2 Place all the remaining ingredients except the mint in a large bowl. Add the dressing and toss to mix. Cover and marinate at room temperature for 2 hours.

3 Toss the salad once again, garnish with the mint, and serve.

TAKE A CHANCE:

- Use fresh dill or oregano instead of the mint.
- Use another variety of rice.
- Add ½ cup diced red bell pepper for color.
- Add a chopped hard-boiled egg.

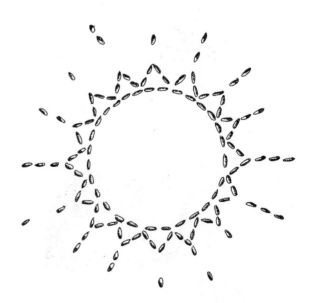

Lemon Lover's Tabbouleh

This salad makes a wonderful one-dish meal during the long, hot summer. It also performs well as an appetizer at parties.

1 cup bulgur wheat

1 cup boiling water

juice of 1½ medium lemons

2 tablespoons extra virgin olive oil

3 large garlic cloves, finely minced

4 scallions, coarsely chopped

2 large tomatoes, seeded and diced

1 large cucumber, peeled, seeded, and coarsely chopped

½ cup finely chopped fresh parsley

¼ teaspoon freshly ground black pepper

½ cup finely chopped fresh mint

½ medium lemon, thinly sliced

SERVES: 4   PREPARATION TIME: 1¼ HOURS

1 Mix the bulgur, boiling water, lemon juice and oil in a large bowl. Cover and let stand at room temperature for 30 minutes, or until the liquid has been absorbed.

2 Add all the remaining ingredients except the mint and lemon slices, and toss well. Adjust the seasonings and toss again. Cover the bowl loosely with plastic wrap and refrigerate for 30 minutes.

3 Stir the mint leaves into the salad, garnish with the lemon slices, and serve immediately.

TAKE A CHANCE:

● Use light sesame or safflower oil instead of the olive oil.

● Substitute cooked buckwheat, barley, or small pasta shells for the bulgur wheat and omit the boiling water.

● Use fresh basil instead of the mint.

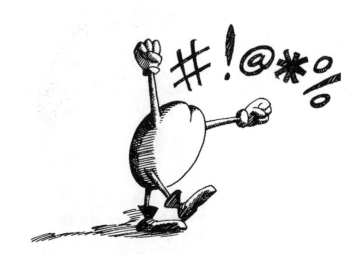

Spicy Buckwheat Salad

The earthy taste of buckwheat is a perfect complement to the light, summery taste of corn, tomatoes, and, of course, lemon.

Dressing

grated zest and juice of 1 medium lemon

2 tablespoons light sesame or safflower oil

$\frac{1}{4}$ teaspoon freshly ground black pepper

Salad

3 scallions, sliced

1 large tomato, seeded and finely chopped

8 ounces mushrooms, sliced

1 cup frozen green peas, thawed

1 cup frozen corn, thawed

1 large red or green jalapeño pepper, seeded and diced

1 cup cooked buckwheat (kasha)

$\frac{1}{4}$ cup finely chopped fresh parsley

SERVES: 4   PREPARATION TIME: 2$\frac{1}{2}$ HOURS

1 Make the dressing by whisking together the lemon zest, lemon juice, oil, and black pepper in a small bowl. Set aside.

2 Place all the remaining ingredients except the parsley in a large bowl. Add the dressing and mix well. Cover and refrigerate for at least 2 hours.

3 Toss the salad once again, garnish with the parsley, and serve immediately.

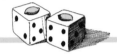

TAKE A CHANCE:

- Use cilantro instead of the parsley.
- Use barley or bulgur wheat instead of the buckwheat.
- Add ½ cup chopped celery.
- Add 1 small finely chopped cucumber.
- Use Thai peppers instead of the jalapeños.

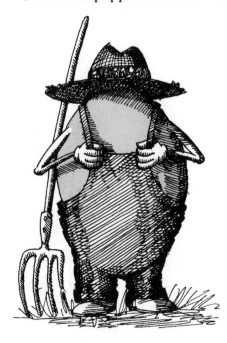

Spicy Soba Noodle Salad

This recipe seems to include a lot of ingredients, but it's really easy to prepare.

Dressing

2 teaspoons canola, safflower, or sunflower oil

3 large red or green jalapeño peppers, seeded and finely minced

3 tablespoons grated fresh ginger

2 large garlic cloves, minced

juice of 1 medium lemon

1 teaspoon toasted sesame oil

1 tablespoon shoyu or tamari sauce

Salad

12 ounces soba (buckwheat) noodles, cooked, drained, and rinsed

2 scallions, cut into matchstick-size pieces

1 cup shredded cabbage

1 medium cucumber, peeled, seeded and coarsely chopped

1 large carrot, peeled and grated

grated zest of 1 medium lemon

$\frac{1}{4}$ cup coarsely chopped peanuts

$\frac{1}{4}$ cup coarsely chopped fresh mint

$\frac{1}{4}$ cup coarsely chopped fresh cilantro

SERVES: 4   PREPARATION TIME: $1\frac{1}{2}$ HOURS

1 To make the dressing, heat the canola, safflower, or sunflower oil in a small saucepan and lightly sauté the jalapeños, ginger, and garlic for 2 to 3 minutes. Remove from the heat and add the lemon juice, sesame oil, and shoyu or tamari sauce. Cool the dressing at room temperature for at least 1 hour.

2 Place the noodles, scallion, cabbage, cucumber, and carrot in a large serving bowl. Add the dressing and toss to mix.

3 Garnish the salad with the lemon zest, peanuts, mint, and cilantro, and serve immediately.

TAKE A CHANCE:

- Use another pasta instead of the soba noodles.
- Add 2 to 3 tablespoons coconut milk to the dressing.
- Add cayenne pepper to the dressing.
- Leave the seeds in the peppers to make the dressing very hot.
- Add strips of red, yellow, or green bell peppers, blanched snow peas, or bean sprouts to the salad.
- Use lemon mint instead of the regular mint.
- Top the salad with toasted coconut.
- Add lemongrass to the dressing.

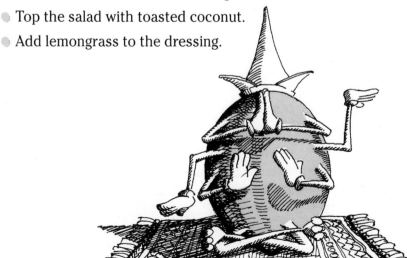

Farfalle Salad With Lemon Mint Dressing

This salad is perfect for a buffet table or as a main meal served with fresh fruit and crusty Italian bread. Dried mint doesn't have much flavor, so use fresh leaves.

Dressing

juice of 2 medium lemons

1 large garlic clove, crushed

1 tablespoon safflower oil

1 cup coarsely chopped fresh mint leaves

$\frac{1}{2}$ teaspoon chopped fresh oregano, or $\frac{1}{4}$ teaspoon dried

$\frac{1}{4}$ teaspoon freshly ground black pepper

Salad

1 medium cucumber, peeled, seeded, and coarsely chopped

1 large tomato, seeded and coarsely chopped

1 medium green bell pepper, seeded and diced

1 pound whole grain farfalle pasta (bow ties), cooked, drained, rinsed, and cooled

SERVES: 4   PREPARATION TIME: 30 MINUTES

1 Make the dressing by combining the lemon juice, garlic, and oil in a small bowl. Add the mint, oregano, and black pepper, and mix thoroughly. Set aside.

2 Combine the vegetables and farfalle in a large serving bowl. Add the dressing, mix well, and serve.

TAKE A CHANCE:

- Use medium-sized shell pasta instead of the farfalle.
- Use a red, yellow, or orange bell pepper instead of the green pepper.
- Add 1 or 2 finely chopped red or green jalapeño peppers.
- Add 1 teaspoon grated lemon zest.
- Use basil instead of the mint.

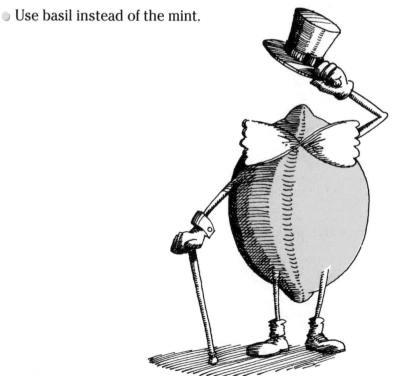

Zesty Tofu With Pasta and Peas

This is a quick-and-easy one-dish meal. Take it on a picnic and serve it with crusty rolls and some fruit. Delicious!

1 pound whole grain tubular pasta such as penne or rigatoni

2 teaspoons safflower oil

1 large carrot, peeled and grated

1 shallot, finely minced

½ cup green peas, blanched 2 to 3 minutes

6 ounces firm tofu, drained and cut into ¼-inch cubes

½ cup Lemon Honey Vinaigrette (see page 218)

¼ teaspoon freshly ground black pepper

SERVES: 4   PREPARATION TIME: 45 MINUTES

1 Cook the pasta in a large pot of boiling water until al dente (firm to the tooth), about 10 to 12 minutes. Drain the pasta, place it in a large bowl, and add the oil, tossing to coat. Cool to room temperature, stirring occasionally to prevent sticking.

2 Add the carrot, shallot, peas, and tofu to the pasta and mix.

3 Add the Lemon Honey Vinaigrette and pepper, and toss well. Serve at room temperature, or chill and serve cold.

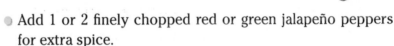

TAKE A CHANCE:

● Add 1 or 2 finely chopped red or green jalapeño peppers for extra spice.

● Add shredded fresh basil.

● Steam the vegetables and warm the Lemon Honey Vinaigrette before mixing with the hot pasta.

● Add the peas to the pasta 2 to 3 minutes before it's done and avoid washing that extra pot!

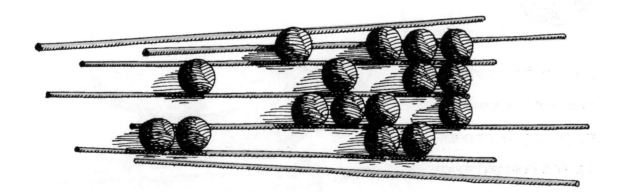

Crunchy Lemon Sandwiches

These tasty sandwiches are a nice change of pace for a light lunch. Crustless and cut in quarters, they're just right for a formal afternoon tea.

3 ounces silken tofu, drained

8 slices whole grain bread

1 tablespoon hulled sunflower seeds

1 medium lemon, peeled, sliced paper thin, and seeded

1 medium cucumber, peeled and sliced paper thin

1 medium carrot, grated

10 red radishes, grated

$\frac{1}{8}$ teaspoon freshly ground black pepper (optional)

$\frac{1}{4}$ cup alfalfa sprouts

SERVES: 4   PREPARATION TIME: 30 MINUTES

1 In a small bowl, mash the tofu with a spoon until creamy. Spread the tofu evenly on 4 of the bread slices and sprinkle with half of the sunflower seeds.

2 Arrange the lemon slices over the tofu and top with the cucumber slices. Spread the grated carrot and red radish over the sandwiches and add the remaining sunflower seeds. Sprinkle with the pepper and alfalfa sprouts.

3 Top the sandwiches with the remaining slices of bread, cut each sandwich into halves or quarters, and serve.

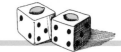

TAKE A CHANCE:

● Add thin slices of tomato.

● Use grated zucchini instead of the cucumber.

● Use chopped walnuts instead of the sunflower seeds.

● Add grated lemon zest to the tofu.

● Use cream cheese, Lemony Yogurt Cheese Spread (see page 236), or Spicy Crushed Chickpeas (see page 56) instead of the tofu.

● Add shredded leaves of regular or lemon mint.

Lemonaid

Some naturalists say that lemon juice helps suppress your appetite if taken before a meal.

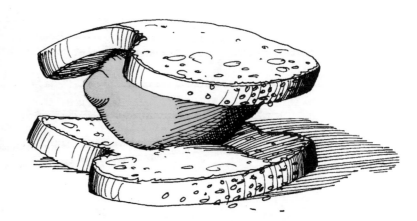

Lemony Vegetable Pita

These pita pockets have the goodness of garden fresh vegetables with the special added attraction of a lemony dressing.

grated zest and juice of 1 medium lemon

$\frac{1}{4}$ cup extra virgin olive oil

$\frac{1}{2}$ teaspoon chopped fresh oregano, or $\frac{1}{4}$ teaspoon dried

$\frac{1}{8}$ teaspoon freshly ground black pepper

1 medium cucumber, peeled and sliced

2 large tomatoes, sliced

1 large zucchini, sliced

1 large green bell pepper, seeded and cut into $\frac{1}{4}$-inch strips

2 pita bread rounds

4 large leaves of red lettuce

$\frac{1}{2}$ cup alfalfa sprouts

SERVES: 4   PREPARATION TIME: 30 MINUTES

1 In a small bowl, mix the lemon zest, lemon juice, oil, oregano, and black pepper. Set aside.

2 Place the cucumber, tomato, zucchini, and green pepper in a large dish and pour the dressing on top. Mix, cover, and marinate for 15 to 20 minutes in the refrigerator.

3 Cut the pita rounds in half. Put a lettuce leaf and a fourth of the vegetable mixture in each pocket. Garnish each sandwich with alfalfa sprouts and serve.

TAKE A CHANCE:

● Add slices of red bell pepper.

● Try adding grated carrot.

● Add some dill, lemon basil, or lemon mint.

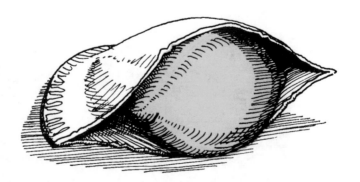

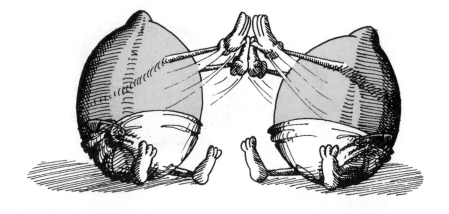

Chapter 5

Soups—
A Soupçon of Lemon

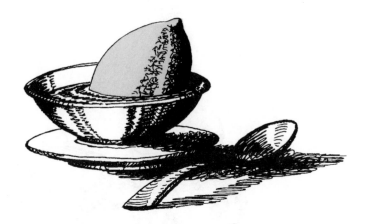

Hot or cold, soup always benefits from the addition of a drop of bright, lemony sunshine. Some of the soups offered here are variations of classics. Others are our own creations.

Lemon Vegetable Broth

This broth is the base for many of the soups presented in this book—or you can use your own favorite broth recipe. Satisfying and nourishing, Lemon Vegetable Broth can also be served by itself. Try it on a winter day in a hand-and-nose-warming mug.

1 medium onion, peeled and left whole

1 teaspoon canola oil

1 large garlic clove, quartered

8 cups water

1 small carrot, peeled and quartered

1 small celery stalk with leaves

2 medium potatoes, peeled and diced

6 whole black peppercorns

juice of 1 medium lemon

SERVES: 6   PREPARATION TIME: 1½ HOURS

1 In a large pot, sauté the onion in the oil for 2 minutes. Add the garlic and continue sautéing for another minute. Add all the remaining ingredients except the lemon juice and simmer for 1 hour.

2 Using a slotted spoon, remove the vegetables (save for another use, if desired). Add the lemon juice to the remaining broth and simmer for 5 minutes. Serve immediately, or use in another recipe.

TAKE A CHANCE:

● Add 1 chopped leek.

● Omit the carrot for a less sweet broth.

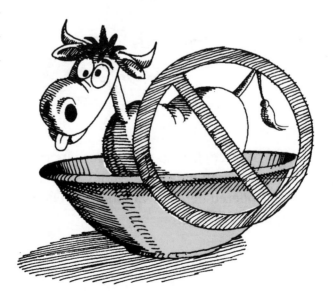

Chinese Lemon Broth With Snow Peas

This recipe is the best of all worlds—simple, elegant, and mysterious.

4 cups Lemon Vegetable Broth (see page 86)

8 ounces silken tofu, drained and cut into ½-inch cubes

zest of 1 medium lemon, slivered

4 ounces snow peas, trimmed

4 cilantro sprigs

SERVES: 4   PREPARATION TIME: 15 MINUTES

1 Place the broth in a large pot and bring to a boil over high heat. Lower the heat, add the tofu, and simmer for 2 minutes. Remove the pan from the heat and stir in the lemon zest and snow peas.

2 Ladle the soup into bowls, garnish with the cilantro, and serve immediately.

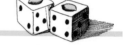

TAKE A CHANCE:

● Add 2 chopped scallions.

● Soak a dried black mushroom in boiling water for about 20 minutes, cut into slivers, and add to the soup.

● Garnish with chopped fresh lemon balm.

Lemonaid

Lemons can be used as a deodorizer in the garbage disposal. Just make them the last thing you grind after cleaning the kitchen.

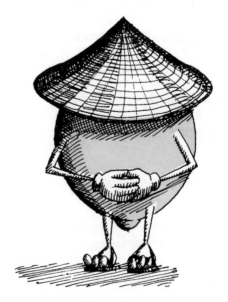

Soothing Lemon Parsley Broth

ven the ancient Greeks used lemon and parsley to dress up their meals. Today, this perfect combination turns a simple broth into a lovely lemony treat. Try it as the first course at your next dinner party.

4 cups Lemon Vegetable Broth (see page 86)

juice of 1 medium lemon

$\frac{1}{2}$ cup chopped fresh parsley

$\frac{1}{2}$ medium lemon, thinly sliced

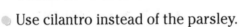

SERVES: 4   PREPARATION TIME: 10 MINUTES

1 Heat the broth in a large pot for 5 minutes over medium heat. Add the lemon juice and parsley, and simmer for 5 minutes.

2 Ladle the broth into bowls, garnish with the lemon slices, and serve immediately.

TAKE A CHANCE:

- Use cilantro instead of the parsley.

- Add a dried red chili pepper to the broth while it is heating. Discard the pepper before serving the broth.

Lemonaid

Citric acid is derived from lemon juice and is used commercially to preserve all kinds of your favorite foods.

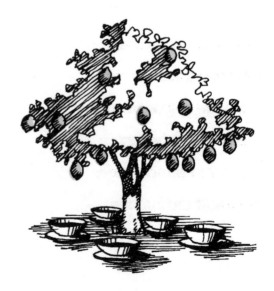

Lemon Minestrone

G et the goodness of fresh vegetables and lemons all in one place. This tends to be a thick soup, but you can use more broth or fewer vegetables for a thinner soup.

8 cups Lemon Vegetable Broth (see page 86)

1 medium onion, coarsely chopped

1 large carrot, peeled and sliced

1 large tomato, peeled, seeded and coarsely diced

2 medium potatoes, peeled and finely diced

2 medium celery stalks, sliced (leaves optional)

1 cup small whole grain macaroni shells

½ cup cooked chickpeas

grated zest of 1 medium lemon

SERVES: 6   PREPARATION TIME: 1 HOUR

1 Heat the broth in a large pot for 5 minutes over medium heat. Add the vegetables and simmer for 25 minutes. Add the macaroni and simmer for 5 more minutes. Add the chickpeas and simmer until the macaroni is done. Neither the vegetables nor the macaroni should be mushy.

2 Add the lemon zest, stir, and serve immediately.

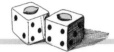

TAKE A CHANCE:

- Use barley or rice instead of the macaroni.
- Garnish with chopped fresh parsley or cilantro.
- Add 8 ounces quartered mushrooms.
- Omit the lemon zest and garnish with chopped fresh lemon balm instead.

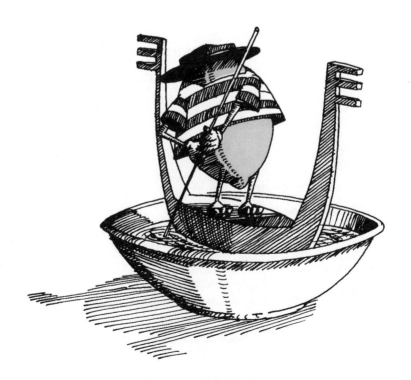

Cold Beet Soup With Zest

Served cold, this Russian take on gazpacho is surprisingly refreshing when the weather is sultry outside. Served hot, this soup is a wonderful borscht on freezing winter days.

5 large beets, stems removed

10 cups water

grated zest and juice of 1 medium lemon

1 tablespoon apple cider vinegar

2 teaspoons date sugar

1 large garlic clove, finely minced

4 scallions, coarsely chopped

3 large potatoes, peeled, boiled, and diced

2 large cucumbers, peeled, seeded, and diced

1 medium green bell pepper, seeded and diced

1 bunch red radishes, coarsely chopped

$\frac{1}{4}$ cup chopped fresh parsley

3 tablespoons chopped fresh dill, or 1$\frac{1}{2}$ tablespoons dried

$\frac{1}{4}$ teaspoon freshly ground black pepper

SERVES: 6   PREPARATION TIME: 3$\frac{1}{2}$ HOURS

1 Place the beets and water in a large pot and bring to a boil over high heat. Reduce heat to medium and simmer until the beets are tender but firm, about 20 minutes. Skim any foam from the cooking liquid. Using a slotted spoon, remove the beets and drain, allowing the cooking water to remain in the pot.

2 When the beets have cooled, use your fingers or a vegetable peeler to remove the skins. Coarsely chop the beets and set aside.

3 Stir the lemon juice, vinegar, and date sugar into the cooking water and simmer for 10 minutes. Return the beets to the pot and simmer for 5 minutes. Remove the soup from the heat, cool, cover, and refrigerate for 3 hours.

4 Mix together all the remaining ingredients except the lemon zest and place an equal amount of the mixture into each soup bowl. Ladle the soup over the vegetables, garnish with the lemon zest, and serve.

TAKE A CHANCE:

- Serve with a dollop of Almost Sour Cream (see page 234).
- Add 1 chopped hard-boiled egg.

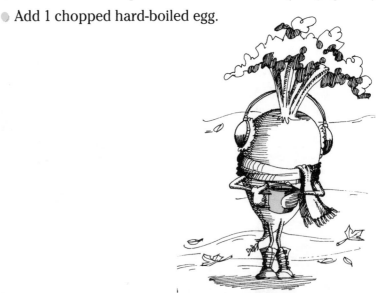

Lemon Strawberry Surprise

A refreshing chilled soup that is terrific for those dog days of summer. And you won't have to heat up the kitchen to make it!

2 pints strawberries, hulled

grated zest and juice of 1 medium lemon

1 cup sparkling mineral water

lemon mint leaves

SERVES: 4   PREPARATION TIME: 2 HOURS

1 Slice 6 of the strawberries and set them aside.

2 Place the lemon zest, lemon juice, and remaining strawberries in a blender or food processor and pulse until the mixture is smooth. Pour into a medium-sized bowl, cover, and refrigerate for about 1 hour.

3 Add the sparkling mineral water to the strawberry mixture, blend well, cover, and refrigerate for another 20 minutes.

4 Ladle the soup into chilled bowls, garnish with the sliced strawberries and the lemon mint, and serve immediately.

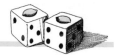

TAKE A CHANCE:

- Use raspberries instead of the strawberries.
- Garnish with regular mint instead of the lemon mint.

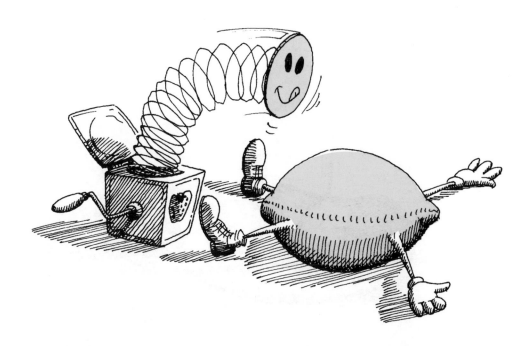

*L*emon-Flecked Cream of Carrot Soup

This is a delicate, creamy soup with flecks of lemon peeking out from every spoonful.

4 cups Lemon Vegetable Broth (see page 86)

3 cups sliced carrots

grated zest and juice of 1 medium lemon

$\frac{1}{4}$ teaspoon freshly ground black pepper

$\frac{1}{4}$ cup silken tofu, mashed

1 tablespoon chopped fresh lemon thyme, or 1$\frac{1}{2}$ tablespoons dried

SERVES: 4   PREPARATION TIME: 30 MINUTES

1 Heat the broth in a large pot for 5 minutes over medium heat. Add the carrots, lemon juice, and pepper, and simmer for 20 minutes, or until the carrots are tender.

2 Place the lemon zest, the broth mixture, and the tofu in a blender or food processor and purée until smooth. If the soup is too thick, add more broth. Return the soup to the pot and heat through.

3 Ladle the soup into bowls, garnish with the lemon thyme, and serve immediately.

TAKE A CHANCE:

- Use dill or regular thyme instead of the lemon thyme.
- Add 2 to 3 sliced leeks when cooking the carrots.
- Instead of incorporating the silken tofu into the soup, serve it in a bowl on the side.
- Omit the lemon thyme and garnish with lemon slices.

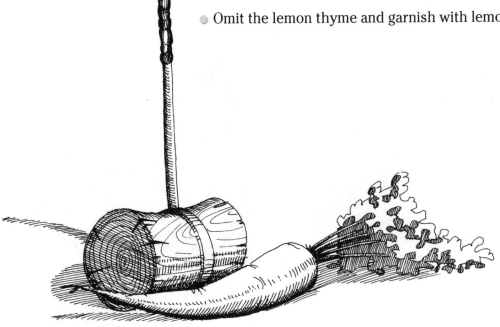

Tangy Tomato Soup

*P**lan to make this soup in the summer when you have garden-fresh tomatoes. You can also use frozen tomatoes.*

8 large tomatoes

grated zest and juice of 1 medium lemon

3 large garlic cloves, finely chopped

½ cup coarsely chopped onion

¼ cup chopped fresh basil

¼ teaspoon freshly ground black pepper

2 cups Lemon Vegetable Broth (see page 86)

3 tablespoons finely chopped fresh cilantro

SERVES: 4   PREPARATION TIME: 45 MINUTES

1 Peel the tomatoes by dipping them briefly in hot water and then removing the peel with a knife. Coarsely chop the tomatoes.

2 In a medium-sized bowl, combine the tomato, lemon juice, garlic, onion, basil, and black pepper. Transfer to a blender or food processor and purée until smooth.

3 Place the puréed mixture in a large pot, add the broth, and blend well. Bring to a boil over high heat, then reduce the heat to medium and simmer for 30 minutes.

4 Ladle the soup into bowls, garnish with the lemon zest and cilantro, and serve immediately.

TAKE A CHANCE:

● Add a few drops of hot sauce before serving.

● Serve with a dollop of plain nonfat yogurt.

● Garnish with lemon slices instead of the zest.

Lemonaid

The outer skin of the lemon can be called the "peel," "rind," or "zest."

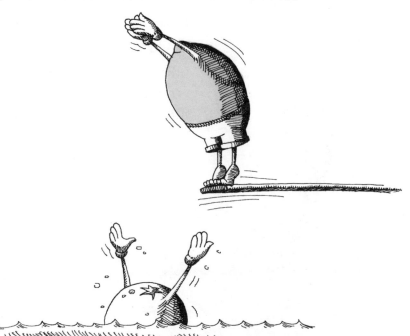

Zestful Zucchini Soup With Basil

If you grow zucchini in your garden, you'll love this terrific soup. It's a great way to use up that always abundant crop. Plus, this soup is easy to make, good for you, and delicious. What more could anyone want?

1 teaspoon canola oil

1 medium onion, coarsely chopped

1 large garlic clove, minced

4 medium zucchinis, cut into ½-inch slices

1½ cups Lemon Vegetable Broth (see page 86)

1 cup water

¼ teaspoon freshly ground black pepper

1 cup chopped fresh basil

grated zest and juice of 1 medium lemon

SERVES: 4   PREPARATION TIME: 30 MINUTES

1 Heat the oil in a large skillet and sauté the onion over low heat until softened, about 3 minutes. Add the garlic and sauté for another minute. Add the zucchini and cook for 5 minutes, stirring occasionally.

2 Add the broth, water, and pepper to the zucchini mixture and cook until the zucchini is tender. Stir in the basil and lemon juice, and simmer for another minute.

3 Place the soup in a blender or food processor in batches and purée until smooth.

4 Reheat the soup or chill in the refrigerator, if desired, then ladle into bowls, garnish with the lemon zest, and serve. This soup can be served warm, at room temperature, or ice cold.

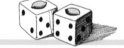

TAKE A CHANCE:

- Use lemon basil instead of the lemon juice.
- Use 1 chopped scallion instead of the regular onion.
- Add a drop or two of hot sauce before serving.
- For chunky-style soup, allow some of the zucchini to remain in slices instead of puréeing it all with the soup.
- Make the soup creamy by adding ½ cup soymilk.

Spirited Black Bean Soup

There is no such thing as a bad black-bean recipe. The spices in this soup are enhanced by the addition of our favorite citrus fruit.

2 cups water

1 cup dried black beans, sorted and rinsed

2 tablespoons light sesame or safflower oil

1 large onion, finely chopped

2 large garlic cloves, minced

juice of 1 medium lemon (reserve the lemon hulls)

3 large red or green jalapeño peppers, finely chopped

2 tablespoons chili powder

3 cups Lemon Vegetable Broth (see page 86)

2 large tomatoes, diced

$\frac{1}{4}$ teaspoon freshly ground black pepper

$\frac{1}{4}$ cup chopped fresh cilantro

SERVES: 4   PREPARATION TIME: 3 HOURS

1 Bring the water to a boil in a large pot and add the beans. Lower the heat and simmer until the beans are tender, about 1½ to 2 hours. Drain the beans and set aside.

2 Heat the oil in a large pot and sauté the onion for about 2 minutes. Add the garlic and sauté for another minute.

3 Cut the juiced lemon hulls into wide strips, add to the onion mixture along with the jalapeños and chili powder, and sauté for 1 minute. Add the lemon juice, broth, beans, tomatoes, and black pepper, and simmer for 30 minutes.

4 Remove and discard the lemon strips. Ladle the soup into bowls, garnish with the cilantro, and serve immediately.

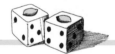

TAKE A CHANCE:

● Use pinto beans instead of the black beans.

● Add 1 teaspoon cayenne pepper for some extra fire.

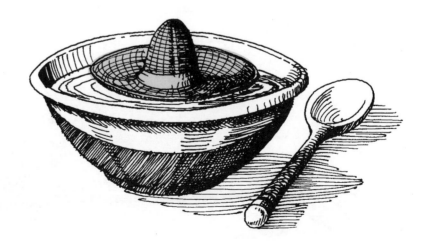

Fresh Pea Soup With Lemon Garlic Croutons

ased on a classic French soup, this recipe can be made with frozen peas. But try making this wonderful dish in the summer, when flavorful fresh peas are available.

1 teaspoon light sesame or safflower oil

1 small white onion, chopped

1 medium leek, white part only, chopped

3 cups Lemon Vegetable Broth (see page 86)

2 cups water

juice of 1 medium lemon

4 cups green peas

Lemon Garlic Croutons (see page 225)

SERVES: 4   PREPARATION TIME: 45 MINUTES

1 Heat the oil in a large pot and sauté the onion and leek for 2 minutes. Add the broth and water, and bring to a boil over high heat. Reduce the heat, add the lemon juice and peas, and simmer for 10 minutes.

2 Place the soup in a blender or food processor in batches and purée until smooth. Return to the pot and heat on low for 5 minutes.

3 Ladle the soup into bowls, garnish with the Lemon Garlic Croutons, and serve immediately.

TAKE A CHANCE:

- Add ½ cup chopped fresh mint or 3 tablespoons chopped fresh dill to the blender.

- Mix the zest of 1 lemon with ¼ cup mashed silken tofu and drop a spoonful on top of each serving.

- Omit the croutons and garnish with grated lemon zest.

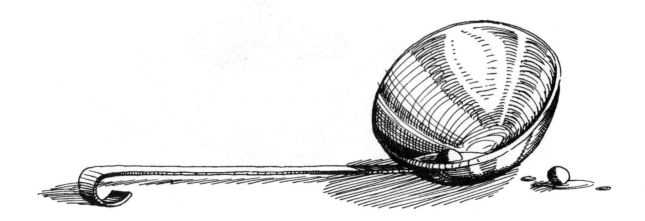

Creamy Lemon Avocado Soup

This creamy soup is very elegant and makes quite an impressive first course for a "natural" gourmet.

2 large avocados, peeled, pitted, and quartered

$\frac{1}{2}$ cup soymilk

grated zest and juice of 1 medium lemon

1 cup Lemon Vegetable Broth (see page 86)

1 teaspoon hot sauce

$\frac{1}{8}$ teaspoon freshly ground black pepper

$\frac{1}{2}$ medium lemon, thinly sliced

2 teaspoons finely chopped fresh cilantro

SERVES: 4   PREPARATION TIME: 20 MINUTES

1 Place the avocados in a blender or food processor and pulse until smooth. Slowly add the soymilk, pulsing only until the ingredients are combined.

2 Pour the avocado mixture into a large pot. Add the lemon zest, lemon juice, broth, hot sauce, and pepper, mixing well. Warm over low heat just long enough to take the chill out of the ingredients. If too thick, add more broth.

3 Ladle the soup into bowls and garnish with the lemon slices and cilantro. This soup can be served warm, at room temperature, or cold.

TAKE A CHANCE:

- Garnish with additional grated lemon zest.
- Omit the lemon zest and garnish with some chopped fresh lemon balm.
- Use mint instead of the cilantro.
- Leave some chunks of avocado in the soup when blending.

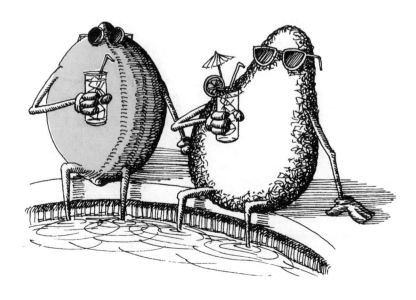

Greek Lemon Soup

The lemony taste of this favorite soup will keep you asking for "just one more bowl, please."

8 cups Lemon Vegetable Broth (see page 86)

3 cups cooked rice

juice of 2 medium lemons

1 large egg

½ medium lemon, sliced

1 tablespoon minced fresh parsley

SERVES: 4   PREPARATION TIME: 25 MINUTES

1 Place the broth in a large pot and bring to a boil over high heat. Reduce the heat and simmer for 5 minutes. Add the rice and simmer again for 5 minutes.

2 Mix the lemon juice and egg together in a small bowl. Slowly add 2 cups of the hot broth to the egg, beating constantly. Slowly pour the egg mixture into the pot, still stirring constantly. Simmer for 1 to 2 minutes. Do not boil or the broth will curdle.

3 Ladle the soup into bowls, garnish with the lemon slices and parsley, and serve immediately.

Note From a Healthy Lemon:

If you're trying to eliminate cholesterol from your diet, use only the egg white in the soup. Or use an egg substitute.

Lemonaid

Lemons stay fresh for three weeks or more if kept in a plastic bag in the refrigerator but only for a week if kept on the kitchen counter.

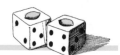

TAKE A CHANCE:

● Try using a very small pasta, such as stars, instead of the rice.

● Add ½ cup grated carrot.

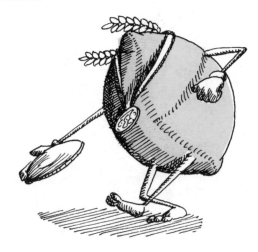

*L*emony Gazpacho

You'll dream of the Spanish hillsides while dining on this wonderfully refreshing soup. It's absolutely perfect for packing in a thermos for a summer picnic. If at home, though, serve plenty of warm tortilla chips on the side.

4 cups tomato juice

2 large garlic cloves, minced

3 large ripe tomatoes, coarsely chopped

1 large cucumber, seeded and coarsely chopped

½ green bell pepper, seeded and coarsely chopped

1 large avocado, peeled, pitted, and thinly sliced

½ large onion, coarsely chopped

1½ cups cooked corn

6 drops hot sauce

juice of 1 medium lemon

¼ teaspoon freshly ground black pepper

2 tablespoons chopped fresh cilantro

SERVES: 4   PREPARATION TIME: 3½ HOURS

1 Place all the ingredients except the cilantro in a large bowl and stir to combine. Cover and refrigerate for 3 hours.

2 Ladle the soup into bowls or mugs, garnish with the cilantro, and serve.

TAKE A CHANCE:

● Add a little grated lemon zest.

● Add some diced red or green jalapeño peppers, chopped zucchini, and/or crookneck squash.

● Increase the amount of hot sauce used or add a few tablespoons of Fresh Lemony Salsa (see page 59).

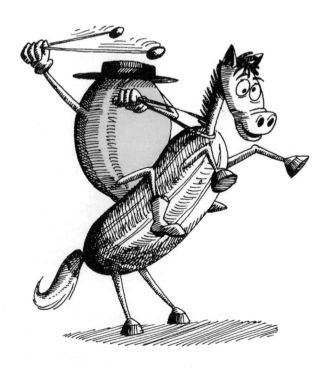

Dried Chili Soup With Lemongrass

Hold onto your tongue! This Thai soup combines hot chilies with cool lemongrass.

1 medium stalk fresh or dried lemongrass

2 large garlic cloves, coarsely chopped

1 teaspoon grated fresh ginger

2 scallions, trimmed and cut into 1-inch pieces

6 small dried red chili peppers, softened in hot water

$\frac{1}{8}$ teaspoon freshly ground black pepper

4 cups Lemon Vegetable Broth (see page 86)

$\frac{1}{2}$ teaspoon chili powder

3 ounces firm tofu, drained and cut into $\frac{1}{2}$-inch cubes

2 tablespoons chopped fresh cilantro

2 scallions, coarsely chopped

SERVES: 4   PREPARATION TIME: 1 HOUR

1 If using fresh lemongrass, finely chop the stalk. If using dried lemongrass, soak the plant in hot water for 2 hours before chopping, then use only the bottom third of the stalk.

2 Place the lemongrass, garlic, ginger, scallion pieces, chilies, and pepper in a blender. Pulse the mixture until a paste forms and set aside. Add a little Lemon Vegetable Broth if the mixture is too dry or sticky.

3 In a large pot, bring the broth to a boil over high heat. Add the lemongrass paste and chili powder, mixing thoroughly. Reduce the heat, add the tofu, and simmer for 10 minutes.

4 Ladle the soup into bowls, garnish with the cilantro and chopped scallions, and serve immediately.

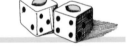

TAKE A CHANCE:

- Use 1½ teaspoons lemon zest instead of the lemongrass.
- Use shallots instead of the scallions.
- Take some of the fire from the soup by removing the seeds from the chilies.

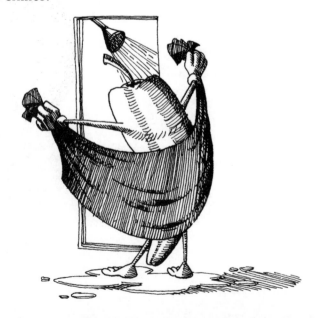

*L*emony Moroccan Harira

*W*e adapted the traditional recipe for Moroccan
Harira by increasing the lentils
and omitting the lamb. This
wonderfully thick soup is warming on a cold winter's night.

1 tablespoon canola oil

½ cup coarsely chopped
celery with leaves

1 large onion, coarsely
chopped

¼ cup chopped fresh
parsley

1 teaspoon ground turmeric

1 teaspoon freshly ground
black pepper

3 large tomatoes, seeded
and coarsely chopped

6 cups Lemon Vegetable
Broth (see page 86)

½ cup dried lentils, sorted
and rinsed

½ cup cooked chickpeas

½ cup fine egg noodles or
whole grain vermicelli

1 large egg

juice of 1 medium lemon

½ medium lemon, thinly
sliced

SERVES: 4   PREPARATION TIME: 1½ HOURS

1 Heat the oil in a large pot and sauté the celery, onion, parsley, turmeric, and pepper over moderately low heat for
about 5 minutes, or until the celery and onion wilt. Add the
tomatoes and cook for 15 minutes, stirring occasionally.

2 Add the broth and lentils to the pot, increase the heat to
high, and bring to a boil. Lower the heat and simmer, partly
covered, for 20 minutes. Add the chickpeas and cook for 15
minutes. The lentils should be well cooked but not mushy.

3 Add the egg noodles or vermicelli to the soup and cook for
5 minutes, until al dente.

4 In a small bowl, beat the egg lightly and add the lemon
juice. Add a ladle of the broth to the egg and stir. Pour the
egg mixture gradually into the soup, stirring slowly to
form long strands of egg.

5 Ladle the soup into bowls, garnish with the lemon slices,
and serve immediately.

Note From a Healthy Lemon:

Reduce the cholesterol in the recipe by using only egg
whites or an egg substitute.

TAKE A CHANCE:

- Lightly sprinkle a bit of ground cinnamon over the soup
before serving.

- Add 3 ounces diced tofu.

- Add more lemon, of course!

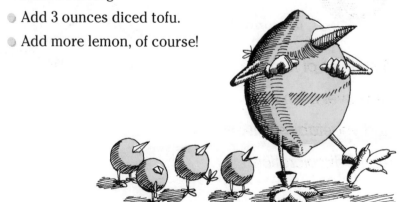

Summer Vegetable Soup

You may feel that summer is not the time to eat a warm soup. But this recipe will show you just how refreshing a bowl of clear lemon broth with fresh vegetables can really be.

6 cups Lemon Vegetable Broth (see page 86)

1 medium carrot, peeled and sliced

½ onion, sliced lengthwise

2 large tomatoes, peeled, seeded, and diced

1 leek, thinly sliced

6 whole black peppercorns

2 avocados, peeled, pitted, and diced

½ medium lemon, thinly sliced

4 cilantro sprigs

SERVES: 4   PREPARATION TIME: 45 MINUTES

1 Heat the broth in a large pot for 5 minutes over medium heat. Add all the remaining ingredients except the avocado, lemon slices, and cilantro, and simmer for 25 minutes, or until the vegetables are barely tender. Add the avocado and lemon slices, and simmer for another 5 minutes.

2 Ladle the soup into bowls, garnish with the cilantro, and serve immediately.

TAKE A CHANCE:

Add 1 finely chopped red or green jalapeño pepper along with the vegetables.

Add 3 ounces diced tofu along with the avocado and lemon.

Dust the soup with ground cinnamon before serving.

Lemonaid

A sprinkle of lemon juice over fresh fruits and vegetables will retard discoloration.

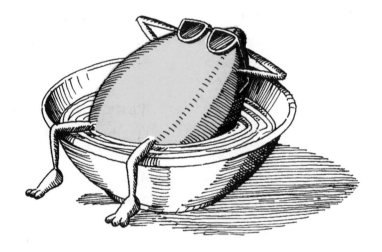

Chicken Noodle Soup With a Drop of Lemon

I f hot chicken soup is the best prescription for what ails you, think of how much better it would be with the goodness of lemons.

1 free-range chicken (about 3 pounds)

juice of 1 medium lemon

1 large celery stalk with leaves

1 large carrot, peeled

1 small onion, peeled and left whole

½ teaspoon Lemon Pepper (see page 227)

2 cups egg noodles

8 thin lemon slices

SERVES: 4   PREPARATION TIME: 9 HOURS

1 Wash the chicken and brush it with the lemon juice.

2 Place the chicken in a large pot and cover with water. Heat to boiling. Reduce the heat to low and skim off any foam.

3 Add the vegetables and Lemon Pepper to the pot, cover, and simmer the soup for 1½ hours, or until the chicken is tender. Transfer the chicken to a large bowl. Remove and discard the vegetables.

4 Cool the broth, cover it, and refrigerate for 6 hours.

5 Remove the skin from the chicken and discard it. Remove the meat from the bones, shred or chop it, and set aside.

6 Skim the fat off the top of the cooled broth. Return to the stove and heat until simmering. Add the chicken pieces and the egg noodles, and simmer for 15 minutes, or until the noodles are tender.

7 Ladle the soup into individual bowls. Squeeze out 2 lemon slices in each bowl, drop in the squeezed slices as garnish, and serve immediately.

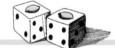

TAKE A CHANCE:

- Use rice instead of the noodles.
- Add ¼ cup chopped fresh parsley or cilantro before serving.
- Add 1 grated carrot along with the meat and noodles.

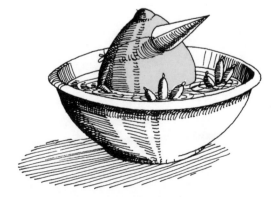

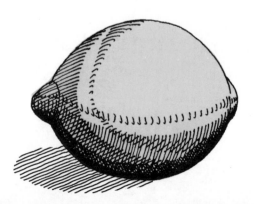

Chapter 6

Vegetarian Main Dishes—
A Little Zest at the End of the Day

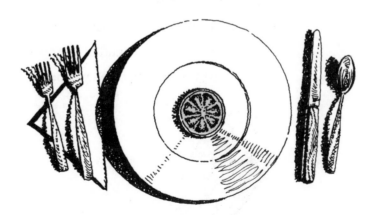

There are very few foods that don't benefit from the addition of lemon in any or all of its faces. Fresh lemon juice, zest, or pulp, and lemon-flavored herbs can all contribute to savory main dishes. The addition of lemon enhances the flavor of the dishes presented in this chapter.

Spaghetti in Uncooked Sauce With a Twist

This is a wonderful way to take advantage of fresh ingredients from the garden when you don't want to spend the whole day making spaghetti sauce.

grated zest and juice of 2 medium lemons

3 medium garlic cloves, coarsely chopped

6 large tomatoes, seeded and coarsely chopped

1 cup thinly sliced fresh basil

2 teaspoons extra virgin olive oil

1 pound thin whole grain spaghetti

$\frac{1}{4}$ teaspoon freshly ground black pepper

SERVES: 4 PREPARATION TIME: 30 MINUTES

1 Combine all the ingredients except the spaghetti and pepper in a small bowl and set aside for 20 minutes.

2 Fill a large pot with water and bring to a full boil. Add the spaghetti and cook until al dente, 8 to 10 minutes. Drain, reserving ¼ cup of the cooking water.

3 Return the spaghetti to the pot and mix with the sauce. Add more lemon juice or some of the reserved cooking water if the pasta seems too dry.

4 Mound the pasta in serving bowls, sprinkle with the pepper, and serve immediately with thick slices of Italian bread.

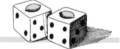

TAKE A CHANCE:

- Use mint instead of the basil.
- Use a tubular pasta instead of the spaghetti.
- Add 1 teaspoon crushed red pepper.

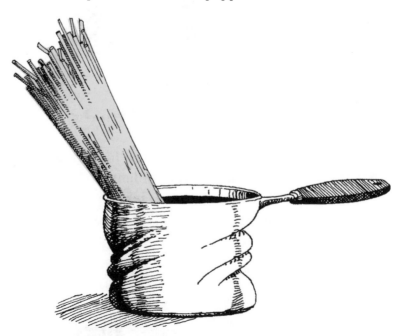

Lemon and Basil on Angel Hair

his is a very delicate dish, without the garlic of an aioli sauce or the cream of an alfredo, but with a wonderful lemony taste.

1 pound whole grain angel hair pasta (capellini)

2 tablespoons soy margarine

4 teaspoons extra virgin olive oil

grated zest and juice of 4 medium lemons

1 cup thinly sliced fresh basil

¼ teaspoon freshly ground black pepper

8 fresh basil leaves

¼ cup freshly grated Parmesan cheese

SERVES: 4   PREPARATION TIME: 15 MINUTES

1 Fill a large pot with water and bring to a full boil. Add the pasta and cook until al dente, 3 to 5 minutes. This pasta cooks very fast, so don't leave the pot unattended too long. Reserve ¼ cup of the cooking water, drain the pasta, and set aside.

2 In a small saucepan, heat the margarine and oil until the margarine has melted. Remove the pan from the heat, add the lemon zest, lemon juice, sliced basil, and pepper, and stir. Return the pasta to the pot and toss with the sauce. If the pasta seems too dry, add some of the reserved cooking water.

3 Mound the pasta on serving plates and garnish with the basil leaves and cheese. Serve with Italian bread and Lemon Antipasto (see page 63).

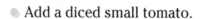

TAKE A CHANCE:

- Add a diced small tomato.
- Use warmed Lemon Vegetable Broth (see page 86) instead of the cooking water if the pasta sticks together.
- Add ½ teaspoon crushed red pepper.
- Use fresh mint instead of the basil.

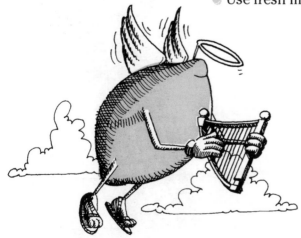

Linguini With Lemony Aioli

Pungent with lemon and fresh garlic, this simple pasta dish is a lemon lover's dream.

1 pound whole grain linguini

juice of 4 medium lemons

8 large garlic cloves, finely minced

$\frac{1}{4}$ cup extra virgin olive oil

$\frac{1}{2}$ teaspoon freshly ground black pepper

SERVES: 4   PREPARATION TIME: 20 MINUTES

1 Fill a large pot with water and bring to a full boil. Add the pasta and cook until al dente, 6 to 8 minutes. Reserve ¼ cup of the cooking water, then drain the pasta and set aside.

2 Return the linguini to the pot, add the remaining ingredients, and toss to combine. If the sauce is too thick or the linguini sticks together, add the reserved cooking water and toss again. Serve immediately with The Perfect Caesar Salad (see page 66).

TAKE A CHANCE:

- Use warmed Lemon Vegetable Broth (see page 86) instead of the cooking water if the linguini sticks together.

- Garnish with bread crumbs sautéed in soy margarine, or with ⅓ cup freshly grated Parmesan cheese.

- Add 1 teaspoon crushed red pepper or 2 teaspoons chopped fresh oregano.

- Halve the amount of ingredients and serve as a first course.

Lemonaid

You can get more juice from a lemon if you let it sit at room temperature and roll it on the counter before you cut it.

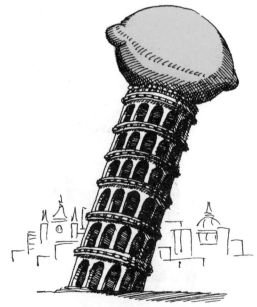

Pasta With Lemon Spinach Pesto

on't wait to have company to serve this easily prepared pasta dish. Your family will thank you for making this special dinner.

SERVES: 4   PREPARATION TIME: 20 MINUTES

½ cup Lemon Vegetable Broth (see page 86)

16 ounces fresh spinach leaves

3 large garlic cloves

juice of 2 medium lemons

⅓ cup pine nuts, toasted

½ cup freshly grated Parmesan cheese

¼ teaspoon freshly ground black pepper

1 pound whole grain linguini

4 fresh basil sprigs

1 medium lemon, cut into wedges

1 Heat 2 tablespoons of the broth in a large skillet and add the spinach. Sauté over medium heat for 2 minutes, or just until the spinach is wilted. Remove the pan from the heat.

2 Place the garlic in a blender or food processor and pulse 3 to 4 times, or until chopped. Add the lemon juice, spinach, pine nuts, cheese, pepper, and remaining broth, and purée until smooth. If the pesto seems too thick, add more lemon juice or broth.

3 Fill a large pot with water and bring to a full boil. Add the linguini and cook until al dente, 6 to 8 minutes. Drain, reserving ¼ cup of the cooking water.

4 Return the linguini to the pot, add the pesto sauce, and toss to combine. If the pasta seems too stiff, add some of the reserved cooking water. Garnish with the basil sprigs and lemon wedges, and serve immediately with crusty rolls.

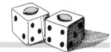

TAKE A CHANCE:

- Use fresh lemon basil or lemon mint instead of the regular basil.
- Use walnuts instead of the pine nuts.
- Add ¼ teaspoon crushed red pepper to the pesto.
- Use fettuccini instead of the linguini.

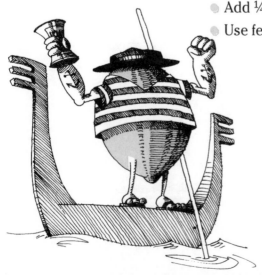

Tart Citrus Vinaigrette Over Linguini

We sometimes get carried away when we make our Tart Citrus Vinaigrette. This recipe is a simple, elegant way to use it. Try not to serve it on salad and pasta on the same night.

1 pound whole grain linguini

1 cup Tart Citrus Vinaigrette (see page 223)

1 cup walnuts

SERVES: 4   PREPARATION TIME: 20 MINUTES

1 Fill a large pot with water and bring to a full boil. Add the pasta and cook until al dente, about 6 to 8 minutes. Drain and return to the pot.

2 Warm the vinaigrette in a small saucepan. Add to the linguini in the pot and mix well.

3 Mound the pasta on serving plates and garnish with the walnuts. Serve immediately with steamed vegetables and breadsticks.

TAKE A CHANCE:

- Garnish with extra lemon and orange zest.
- Add some crushed red pepper to the vinaigrette.

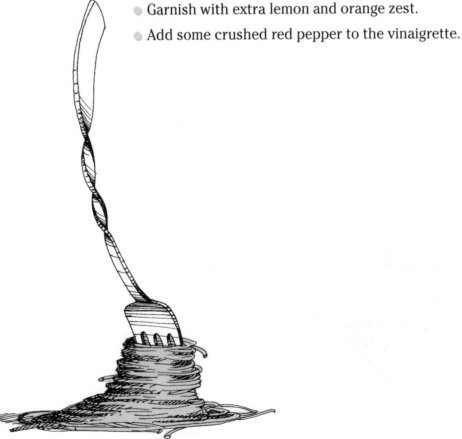

Creamy Lemon Alfredo

This version of Fettuccini Alfredo won't tip your bathroom scale to the plus side because it's much lighter than the classic cream-based version.

16 ounces silken tofu

$\frac{1}{4}$ cup soymilk

$\frac{3}{4}$ cup Lemon Vegetable Broth (see page 86)

grated zest and juice of 1 medium lemon

$\frac{1}{4}$ cup freshly grated Parmesan cheese or tofu-Parmesan cheese

1 pound whole grain fettuccini pasta

SERVES: 4   PREPARATION TIME: 20 MINUTES

1 Place the tofu in a blender or food processor and pulse 3 to 4 times, until creamy. Add the soymilk and blend until the mixture is smooth. Set aside.

2 In a large saucepan, warm the broth over medium heat. Stir in the lemon zest, lemon juice, tofu mixture, and 2 tablespoons of the cheese. Reduce the heat to low and cook for 3 minutes, stirring occasionally. Add more broth if the sauce is too stiff.

3 Fill a large pot with water and bring to a full boil. Add the pasta and cook until al dente, 6 to 8 minutes. Drain. Add the pasta to the saucepan and toss with the sauce.

4 Mound the pasta on serving plates and garnish with the remaining cheese. Serve immediately with crusty rolls and Romaine With Olive Oil and Lemon (see page 65).

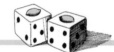

TAKE A CHANCE:

- Add ½ cup chopped walnuts.
- Stir in ½ cup minced parsley or cilantro.
- Add 1 cup cooked peas.

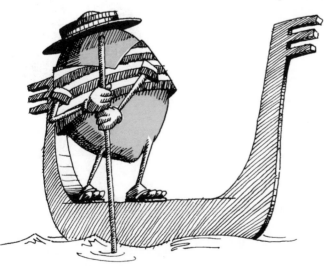

Pasta With Lemon Chili Sauce

Serve this chunky sauce over a tubular pasta such as penne or rigatoni. The lemon- and chili-flecked tomatoes will hide inside the tubes and surprise your mouth as you bite down.

1 tablespoon extra virgin olive oil

¼ cup finely chopped onion

3 large garlic cloves, minced

grated zest and juice of 2 medium lemons

4 large dried red chili peppers, crushed, or 2 teaspoons crushed red pepper

4 large tomatoes, seeded and diced

1 pound whole grain tubular pasta such as penne or rigatoni

¼ cup chopped fresh cilantro

SERVES: 4   PREPARATION TIME: 20 MINUTES

1 Heat the oil in a large skillet and sauté the onion and garlic for 1 minute. Add the lemon zest, lemon juice, and chili peppers, and sauté for 1 more minute. Stir in the tomatoes and cook over medium heat for 5 minutes.

2 Fill a large pot with water and bring to a full boil. Add the pasta and cook until al dente, 10 to 12 minutes. Drain.

3 Place the pasta and the sauce in a large bowl, mix well, and garnish with the cilantro. Serve immediately with crusty French bread and Greek Salad With a Lemon Tang (see page 64).

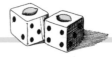

TAKE A CHANCE:

- Use chili powder instead of the red chili peppers or crushed red pepper.

- Add 2 teaspoons chopped fresh oregano or basil.

Lemonaid

You can get rid of the taste of garlic in your mouth by eating a slice of lemon.

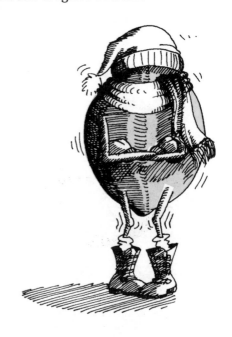

Enchiladas With Zesty Tomatillo Sauce

Tomatillos are Mexican green tomatoes. On their own, they have a slightly bitter taste. Made into a zesty sauce, they will transform your enchiladas into a treat. Olé!

Sauce

1 medium onion, coarsely chopped

3 large garlic cloves, coarsely chopped

1 large red or green jalapeño pepper, seeded and chopped

$\frac{1}{2}$ cup chopped fresh cilantro

24 tomatillos, husks removed and coarsely chopped

2 teaspoons arrowroot

1 cup Lemon Vegetable Broth (see page 86)

juice of 1 medium lemon

juice of 1 large lime

1 teaspoon date sugar

Enchiladas

2 cups firm tofu, drained and cut into $\frac{1}{2}$-inch pieces

$\frac{1}{4}$ cup Almost Sour Cream (see page 234)

2 cups shredded tofu cheese

2 tablespoons chopped fresh cilantro

1 teaspoon chopped fresh oregano, or $\frac{1}{2}$ teaspoon dried

6 medium organic whole wheat tortillas

SERVES: 6   PREPARATION TIME: 45 MINUTES

1 To make the sauce, place the onion, garlic, and jalapeño pepper in a blender or food processor and pulse 2 times. Add the cilantro and pulse once again. Add the tomatillos and pulse until the mixture is smooth.

2 Place the tomatillo mixture in a medium-sized saucepan and simmer for 5 minutes.

3 In a small bowl, stir the arrowroot into 2 tablespoons of the broth until it dissolves. Add along with the remaining broth to the tomatillos and simmer for 10 minutes. Add the citrus juices and date sugar, and simmer for 10 minutes more, or until the sauce starts to thicken.

4 To make the enchilada filling, mix the tofu with the Almost Sour Cream, half of the tofu cheese, the cilantro, and the oregano in a small bowl. Set aside.

5 Soften the tortillas in the microwave for 10 seconds or in a 325°F oven for 1 minute. Divide the filling among the tortillas and roll each tortilla around the filling. Place the enchiladas seam side down in one layer in an oiled baking dish.

6 Pour the tomatillo sauce over the tortillas, cover with foil, and bake in a 350°F oven for 15 minutes. Uncover, sprinkle with the remaining tofu cheese, and bake for 15 more minutes, or until the cheese has melted.

7 Serve immediately with extra sauce and sour cream.

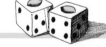

TAKE A CHANCE:

● Add 1 tablespoon grated lemon zest to the enchilada filling.

● Use your favorite meat substitute instead of the tofu.

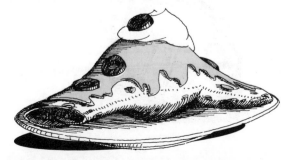

*F*iesta Burros With Black Beans

A burro is a large burrito—an old Mexican standard that includes just about anything rolled up in a tortilla. Wonderful warm or cold, these bean-salad burros are great on picnics or whenever appetites are large but time is short.

2 cups cooked black beans

grated zest and juice of 2 medium lemons

4 large garlic cloves, crushed

2 large tomatoes, coarsely chopped

1 cup minced fresh parsley

2 teaspoons extra virgin olive oil

$\frac{1}{4}$ teaspoon freshly ground black pepper

4 organic whole wheat tortillas, 12 inches each

$\frac{1}{4}$ cup Almost Sour Cream (see page 234), optional

SERVES: 4   PREPARATION TIME: 20 MINUTES

1 Warm the beans over low heat in a small saucepan until just heated and transfer to a medium-sized mixing bowl. Add the lemon zest, lemon juice, garlic, tomato, and parsley, and mix lightly. Add the olive oil and pepper, and mix well.

2 Soften the tortillas in the microwave for 10 seconds or in a 325°F oven for 1 minute. Do not allow them to dry out.

3 Place about ½ cup of the bean mixture in the middle of each warm tortilla and top with a teaspoon of Almost Sour Cream, if desired. Fold the tortilla around the mixture to form a burrito and serve immediately.

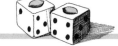

TAKE A CHANCE:

- Add more lemon, garlic, or olive oil to taste.
- Fill pita bread with the bean mixture instead of using the tortillas.
- Add ½ teaspoon dried oregano or 1 teaspoon fresh.
- Place the burros in an ungreased medium-sized baking dish. Cover with aluminum foil and bake at 350°F until the beans are hot in the center of the tortillas, about 5 to 7 minutes.
- Add ¼ teaspoon cayenne pepper for some spice.
- Mince a hard-boiled egg and add to the bean-salad mixture.
- Use cilantro instead of the parsley.
- Top with chopped avocado or Zesty Guacamole (see page 58).

Citrus Vegetable Fajitas

Marinade

juice of 1 medium lemon

juice of 1 medium orange

juice of 1 large lime

l large garlic clove, minced

$\frac{1}{8}$ teaspoon freshly ground black pepper

Fajitas

12 ounces firm tofu, drained and cut into $\frac{1}{2}$-inch cubes

2 tablespoons light sesame or safflower oil

1 medium green bell pepper, seeded and cut into $\frac{1}{4}$-inch strips

1 medium red bell pepper, seeded and cut into $\frac{1}{4}$-inch strips

1 medium yellow bell pepper, seeded and cut into $\frac{1}{4}$-inch strips

2 large Anaheim peppers, seeded and cut into $\frac{1}{4}$-inch strips

2 large red or green jalapeño peppers, seeded and cut into $\frac{1}{8}$-inch strips

1 medium zucchini, cut in half lengthwise and then cut into strips

8 ounces mushrooms, sliced

1 medium onion, cut in half and then cut into thin slices

8 medium organic whole wheat tortillas

Fresh Lemony Salsa (see page 59)

SERVES: 4   PREPARATION TIME: $1\frac{1}{2}$ HOURS

1 To make the marinade, combine all of the marinade ingredients in a medium-sized bowl. Stir in the tofu, cover, and let sit at room temperature for 1 hour.

2 Heat the oil in a large skillet and sauté the vegetables lightly over high heat for 3 minutes. They should be very crisp. Remove the vegetables from the skillet and keep warm in a large dish.

3 Turn the heat down to medium-high and add the tofu and marinade. Sauté for 3 minutes. Return the vegetables to the skillet and cook for 2 minutes more, stirring constantly.

4 Serve the filling immediately with the warm tortillas and the Fresh Lemony Salsa. Instruct your guests to fill their tortillas with the vegetables and tofu, and top with the salsa.

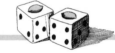

TAKE A CHANCE:

- Add more jalapeños to make the mixture hotter.
- Sprinkle the vegetables with toasted sesame seeds before serving.
- Use crookneck squash instead of the zucchini.
- Add thin slices of lemon when sautéing the vegetables.
- Add broccoli florets to the mixture.
- For a tarter taste, add the juice of 2 more lemons instead of using orange and lime juice.

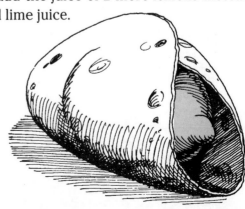

Unbelievable Pizza With Marinated Vegetables and Tofu

What's so unbelievable is that this pizza is good for you. This is a basic recipe— let your imagination go wild!

Crust

1 package dry active yeast

1 tablespoon honey

1 cup lukewarm water

1 cup whole wheat pastry flour

2 tablespoons light sesame or safflower oil

2 cups unbleached flour

Topping

8 ounces firm tofu, drained and cut into $\frac{1}{4}$-inch cubes

2 large tomatoes, seeded and coarsely chopped

$\frac{1}{2}$ large onion, cut into thick rings

3 large garlic cloves, chopped

$\frac{1}{4}$ cup brine-cured black olives, pitted and chopped

grated zest and juice of 1 medium lemon

2 teaspoons extra virgin olive oil

2 teaspoons chopped fresh oregano, or 1 teaspoon dried

1 tablespoon cornmeal

6 ounces feta cheese

SERVES: 4   PREPARATION TIME: $1\frac{1}{2}$ HOURS

1 To prepare the pizza dough, dissolve the yeast and honey in the water in a large bowl. Allow to sit for 5 minutes.

2 Stir the pastry flour and sesame or safflower oil into the yeast mixture. Add the unbleached flour ½ cup at a time, mixing until a soft dough forms. Turn the dough out onto a lightly floured board and knead until smooth and elastic. Add the remaining flour a little at a time until the dough is no longer sticky.

3 Place the dough in a large bowl coated with oil or nonstick spray and turn the dough once so that both sides become coated. Cover and let rise in a warm place until doubled in size, about 45 minutes.

4 While the dough is rising, mix all of the topping ingredients except the cornmeal and cheese in a large bowl and allow to marinate for 30 minutes.

5 Punch the dough down and remove it from the bowl. Cut the dough in half for 2 medium pizzas or in quarters for 4 individual pizzas.

6 Place a ball of dough on a large board covered with cornmeal. Flatten the dough with the heel of your hand, then carefully stretch and pull it to the desired size. Press it into shape on a pizza pan or cookie sheet and, using your fingertips, form a ½-inch rim around the crust. Repeat with the other portions of dough.

7 Divide the topping among the pizzas and spread over the crust. Crumble the feta cheese on top. Bake in a 500°F oven for 10 to 15 minutes, or until the cheese is melted.

8 Remove the pizza from the oven and let stand for 5 minutes before cutting and serving.

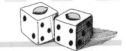

Lemonaid

Make dull copper pots and pans shine by rubbing them with coarse salt and the hulls of squeezed lemons.

TAKE A CHANCE:

- Add 1 teaspoon grated lemon zest to the crust.
- Add mushrooms or zucchini to the vegetable topping.
- Use fresh dill instead of the oregano.
- Crumble on your favorite meat substitute.
- Make the dough for the pizza crust ahead of time and store it in the freezer. To do this, complete steps 1 through 3 of the recipe. Once the dough has doubled in size, punched it down, coat it with cornmeal, wrap it securely in plastic, and place it in the freezer for up to several weeks. When ready, defrost the dough at room temperature for 2 to 3 hours or in the refrigerator overnight. Then follow the recipe again, beginning with step 4.

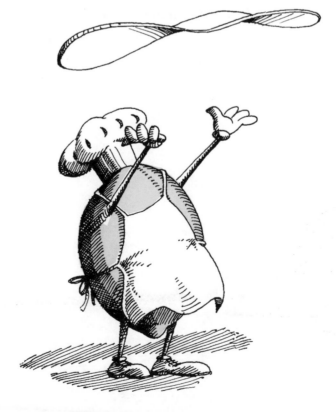

Grilled Tofu With Zesty Barbecue Sauce

When cooking this terrific tofu on your barbecue, put the skewers on a kabob rack. The parallel bars will support the skewers, make it easier to turn the tofu, and keep it from sticking to the grill.

2 cakes (12 ounces each) firm tofu, drained and cut in half

½ cup Zesty Barbecue Sauce (see page 232)

SERVES: 4   PREPARATION TIME: 20 MINUTES

1 Push 2 metal skewers, or 2 long bamboo skewers that have been soaked in water for 20 minutes, through the 4 pieces of tofu.

2 Place the 2 skewers with the 4 pieces of tofu on a hot grill and cook the tofu for 2 minutes on each side. Place 1 tablespoon of barbecue sauce on each piece of tofu and grill for about 5 minutes more on each side, or until the tofu is browned.

3 Arrange the skewers with the tofu on a platter, with the remaining barbecue sauce on the side. Serve with brown rice and steamed vegetables.

TAKE A CHANCE:

- After draining the tofu, sprinkle it with the juice of 1 medium lemon and let it marinate for 30 minutes.

- Instead of grilling, broil the tofu in the oven for 3 to 5 minutes on each side.

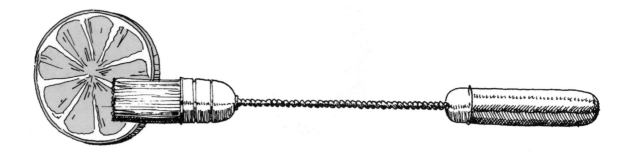

Sautéed Tofu in Lemon Thyme

After a long, hard day, the last thing you want is to play around in the kitchen. This quick and easy tofu dish certainly fits the bill. Nothing could be easier!

2 tablespoons Mock Lemon Butter (see page 235)

¼ cup thinly sliced onion

1 teaspoon chopped fresh lemon thyme, or ½ teaspoon dried

12 ounces firm tofu, drained and cut into ½-inch cubes

1 tablespoon minced fresh cilantro

Lemonaid

A tablespoon of lemon juice mixed with a cup of plain yogurt makes a soothing sunburn cream.

SERVES: 4   PREPARATION TIME: 15 MINUTES

1 Melt the Mock Lemon Butter in a large skillet. Add the onion and sauté for 2 to 3 minutes. Add the lemon thyme and sauté for another minute. Add the tofu and stir-fry until it is golden brown.

2 Place the tofu in a large dish and pour the butter from the pan over the top. Garnish with the cilantro and serve over brown rice with Wilted Citrus Spinach Salad (see page 67) on the side.

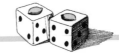

TAKE A CHANCE:

- Use marjoram instead of the lemon thyme.

- Instead of cutting the tofu into cubes, cut it into quarters.

- Marinate the tofu cubes in the juice of l lemon for 30 minutes before sautéing.

- Sauté 1 tablespoon chopped lemongrass or lemon balm in plain soy margarine instead of using the Mock Lemon Butter.

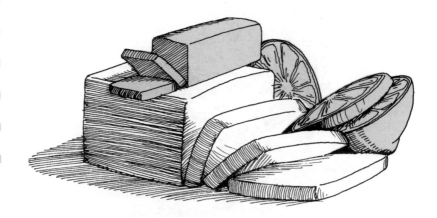

Tofu With Citrus Stuffing

This stuffing will really perk up those ordinary dinners.

½ cup Lemon Vegetable Broth (see page 86)

½ cup chopped onion

grated zest and juice of 1 medium lemon

grated zest and juice of 1 medium orange

1 fresh sage leaf, chopped, or ½ teaspoon dried

1 teaspoon chopped fresh thyme, or ½ teaspoon dried

2 cups whole grain bread cubes

1 pound firm tofu, drained

2 tablespoons chopped fresh parsley

SERVES: 4   PREPARATION TIME: 40 MINUTES

1 Heat 2 tablespoons of the broth in a large skillet and sauté the onion for 2 minutes. Add the citrus zest and juices, the sage and thyme, and the remaining broth, and simmer for 1 minute. Add the bread cubes and stir until evenly moistened. Add more broth if necessary.

2 Using a sharp knife, cut out the center of the tofu, making a pocket and leaving a shell about ½-inch thick. Stuff the pocket with the filling.

3 Place the stuffed tofu in an oiled 1½-quart casserole dish and surround it with any leftover stuffing. Bake in a 350°F oven for 20 minutes, or until the tofu turns light brown.

4 Arrange on a serving plate, garnish with the parsley, and serve with Steamed Vegetable Medley With Lemon and Shoyu (see page 186).

TAKE A CHANCE:

- Use the stuffing in tomatoes or green bell peppers.
- Add some nuts.
- Stuff the tofu with Citrus-Studded Wild Rice (see page 135) instead of the bread mixture.

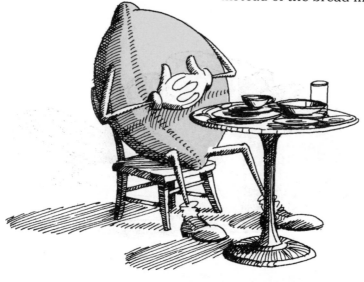

Marinated Tofu Stir-Fry

This is a hearty meal filled with fresh vegetables and some lovely lemon.

Marinade

juice of 1 medium lemon

$\frac{1}{4}$ teaspoon grated fresh ginger

1 tablespoon shoyu or tamari sauce

$\frac{1}{4}$ teaspoon ground cumin

$\frac{1}{4}$ teaspoon freshly ground black pepper

Stir-Fry

12 ounces firm tofu, drained and cut into 1-inch cubes

juice of 1 medium lemon

2 tablespoons shoyu or tamari sauce

1 teaspoon light sesame or safflower oil

1 small onion, sliced

4 thin lemon slices

1 small zucchini, sliced

1 medium carrot, sliced

1 cup broccoli florets

$\frac{1}{4}$ cup finely chopped red bell pepper

$\frac{1}{4}$ cup snow peas, trimmed

$\frac{1}{2}$ cup Lemon Vegetable Broth (see page 86)

1 tablespoon sesame seeds, toasted

SERVES: 4   PREPARATION TIME: 1 HOUR

1 To make the marinade, combine all of the marinade ingredients in a medium-sized bowl. Stir in the tofu, cover, and let stand at room temperature for 45 minutes.

2 Heat the lemon juice, 2 tablespoons shoyu or tamari sauce, and oil in a large skillet. Add the onion and sauté for 2 minutes over medium heat.

3 Discard the marinade and add the tofu to the skillet. Sauté for 2 minutes, or until the tofu is lightly browned. Use a slotted spoon to transfer the tofu to a warmed dish.

4 Add the lemon slices, vegetables, and broth to the skillet and stir-fry over medium heat until the vegetables are cooked but still very crisp. Return the tofu to the pan and cook for an additional 3 minutes.

5 Sprinkle with the toasted sesame seeds and serve over rice or couscous.

TAKE A CHANCE:

- Add the grated zest of 1 lemon to the vegetables.
- Use walnuts or cashews instead of the sesame seeds.
- Steam the vegetables instead of stir-frying them, then mix them with the sautéed tofu.
- Add eggplant or green beans.

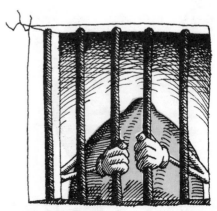

Tofu and Spinach in Phyllo

I n Greece, this dish is called spanakopeta. There are as many spellings of the name of this dish as there are different ways to make it. We've added a touch of lemon and tofu. Just call it "good"!

4 teaspoons extra virgin olive oil

1 cup chopped scallions

1 large garlic clove, minced

2 cups chopped fresh spinach

juice of 1 medium lemon

8 ounces feta cheese, crumbled

½ cup chopped fresh parsley

2 large eggs

8 ounces silken tofu, mashed

¼ teaspoon ground nutmeg

¼ teaspoon freshly ground black pepper

1 tablespoon soy margarine

12 sheets phyllo dough

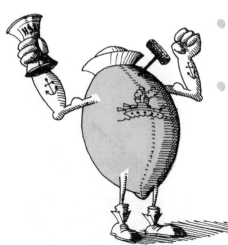

SERVES: 4   PREPARATION TIME: 1 HOUR

1 Heat 1 teaspoon of the oil in a large skillet. Add the scallions and garlic, and sauté for 2 minutes over medium heat. Add the spinach and sauté until it is limp. Remove the skillet from the heat, transfer the spinach mixture to a large bowl, and blend in all the remaining ingredients except the margarine, phyllo dough, and remaining oil. Set aside.

2 Melt the margarine, mix it with the remaining oil, and brush some of the mixture on the bottom and sides of a 9-x-13-inch baking dish. Using 6 sheets of the phyllo, line the baking dish, with the sides of the phyllo overhanging the pan. Brush with more margarine mixture. Spread the spinach mixture over the phyllo and fold the overhanging phyllo over the spinach.

3 Fold the remaining phyllo sheets to fit the pan and lay over the spinach one at a time, brushing each with margarine before adding the next. Brush the top with margarine. Bake in a 350°F oven for 45 minutes, or until golden brown.

4 Immediately cut into squares and serve hot, or cool before cutting and serve at room temperature.

TAKE A CHANCE:

- Add 2 tablespoons fresh dill or 1 tablespoon dried to the spinach mixture.

- In step 2, spread half the spinach mixture in the pan, sprinkle with 2 diced hard-boiled eggs, cover with the remaining spinach, and continue as directed.

- Cut the phyllo into 3-inch-wide strips, brush with the margarine, and place 1 teaspoon of the spinach mixture at the bottom of each strip. Fold to form a triangle, brush the outside with margarine, and bake at 350°F for 20 minutes, or until golden brown. This makes about 50 appetizers.

Baked Tofu Cutlets With Honey and Lemon

I n this dish, the honey-and-lemon marinade turns plain tofu into pure delight, and the lemon slices add tartness to each mouthful.

¼ cup Honey and Lemon Spread (see page 241)

3 tablespoons shoyu or tamari sauce

12 ounces firm tofu, drained

½ medium lemon, thinly sliced

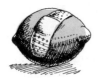

Lemonaid

Grated lemon zest or lemon juice can be used as a substitute for salt in many dishes.

SERVES: 4   PREPARATION TIME: 3 HOURS

1 Mix the Honey and Lemon Spread with the shoyu or tamari sauce in a small bowl and set aside.

2 Cut the drained tofu in half lengthwise to form slabs, then cut each slab in half to form cutlets. Place the cutlets side by side on a large plate. Pour half of the Honey and Lemon Spread over the cutlets, and turn the cutlets so that both sides are covered. Marinate in the refrigerator for 2 hours, turning the tofu at least once.

3 Remove the tofu from the marinade, reserving the marinade for later use. Place the tofu in an oiled 9-x-13-inch baking dish. Arrange the lemon slices on top of the tofu and bake in a 350°F oven for 25 to 30 minutes, or until the tofu is lightly browned.

4 Arrange the tofu on a serving platter. Warm the reserved marinade and pour it over the tofu. Serve with Citrus-Studded Wild Rice (see page 135) and a green salad.

TAKE A CHANCE:

● Omit the shoyu or tamari sauce and add 2 teaspoons chili powder, dried sage, or dried thyme to the Honey and Lemon Spread.

● Top the cooked tofu with finely chopped scallions.

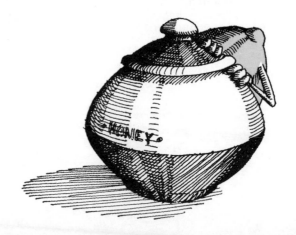

Tofu Stew With Lemons and Olives

An adaptation of a Moroccan stew containing chicken, this vegetarian version is quick and easy to prepare. Serve it over steamed brown basmati rice with plenty of crisp, fresh bread.

4 tablespoons Lemon Vegetable Broth (see page 86)

1 large onion, coarsely chopped

2 large garlic cloves, coarsely chopped

1 cup chopped fresh cilantro

1 teaspoon grated fresh ginger

pinch of saffron, pulverized

12 ounces firm tofu, drained and cut into $\frac{1}{2}$-inch cubes

2 cups water

10 brine-cured olives such as Greek Kalamatas

$\frac{1}{4}$ teaspoon freshly ground black pepper

$\frac{1}{2}$ Moroccan Preserved Lemon (see page 246)

juice of 1 medium lemon

SERVES: 4   PREPARATION TIME: 45 MINUTES

1 Heat the broth in a large skillet over medium heat. Add the onion, garlic, cilantro, ginger, and saffron, and sauté for 3 minutes. Add the tofu and sauté for 2 minutes more. Add the water and bring the mixture to a boil. Reduce the heat to medium-low and simmer for 30 minutes.

2 Using a slotted spoon, transfer the tofu to a serving plate and keep warm. Pour the contents of the skillet into a blender or food processor and purée until smooth.

3 Return the puréed mixture to the skillet. Add the olives, pepper, and preserved lemon, and bring just to a boil, stirring constantly. Remove the skillet from the heat and add the lemon juice. If the broth is too "soupy," mash several pieces of tofu into the broth.

4 Remove the preserved lemon, pour the broth over the warmed tofu, and serve over brown basmati rice.

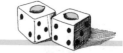

TAKE A CHANCE:

- Add a cinnamon stick to the broth during cooking.
- Use parsley instead of the cilantro.
- Add 1 whole egg or 1 egg white to the blender when puréeing the broth.
- Use the grated zest of 1 lemon instead of the Moroccan Preserved Lemon.

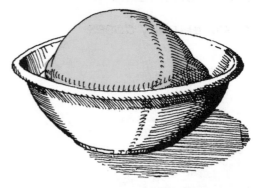

Tofu Smothered in Lemon and Onions

The tart flavor of this dish is not for sissies. Freezing tofu after it is drained and sliced gives it the consistency of chicken.

1 pound firm tofu, drained, sliced, wrapped, and frozen

2 large onions, cut into thin rings

juice of 2 medium lemons

3 large garlic cloves, finely minced

1 teaspoon chili powder

SERVES: 4   PREPARATION TIME: 2 HOURS

1 Fill a medium-sized bowl with boiling water. Place the frozen wrapped tofu in the bowl for 20 to 30 minutes. After it is thawed, unwrap the tofu, place it in a large bowl, and cover with the onions.

2 In a small bowl, mix together the lemon juice, garlic, and chili powder. Pour the mixture over the onions and tofu. Cover and marinate at room temperature for 1 hour, turning occasionally.

3 Transfer the marinade and onions to a small saucepan and cook over medium heat for 10 minutes. Add the tofu to the pan and cook for an additional 2 to 3 minutes, or until the tofu is warmed through.

4 Place the tofu on a large serving dish and smother with the sauce and onions. Serve with Brown Rice Mexican Style (see page 131).

TAKE A CHANCE:

• Instead of heating the tofu cutlets in the marinade, broil them before smothering with the lemon juice and onions.

• Add sliced red or green jalapeño peppers to the onion mixture.

• Use fresh tofu instead of the frozen.

Lemonaid

Cover raw vegetables with lemon juice and store in a jar in the refrigerator for tangy "pickled" treats.

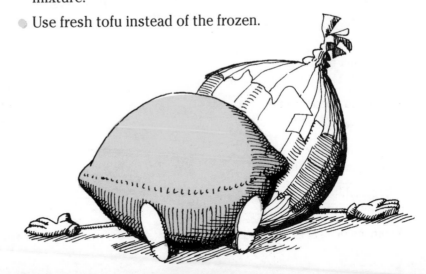

7ofu With Lemongrass and Coconut Curry Sauce

Coconut milk gives this dish a creamy texture without a heavy coconut taste. Use powdered lemongrass only if other forms are not available.

Marinade

3 tablespoons finely chopped fresh or dried lemongrass

3 large garlic cloves, finely minced

3 Thai chili peppers, seeded and finely chopped

$\frac{1}{3}$ cup shoyu or tamari sauce

$\frac{1}{3}$ cup curry paste

1 teaspoon date sugar

Sauce

1 pound tofu, drained and cut into $\frac{1}{2}$-inch cubes

3 tablespoons Lemon Vegetable Broth (see page 86)

2 tablespoons finely chopped fresh or dried lemongrass

2 large garlic cloves, finely minced

3 Thai chili peppers, seeded and finely chopped

14 ounces coconut milk

$1\frac{1}{2}$ cups water

2 sweet potatoes, peeled and cut into $\frac{1}{4}$-inch slices

1 large white onion, cut lengthwise into thin slices

8 ounces rice sticks, cooked

SERVES: 4   PREPARATION TIME: 1$\frac{1}{2}$ HOURS

1 To make the marinade, combine the 3 tablespoons lemongrass and all of the remaining marinade ingredients in a medium-sized bowl. Stir in the tofu, cover, and let stand at room temperature for 1 hour.

2 Heat the broth in a large saucepan. Add the tofu and marinade, and cook over medium heat for 2 minutes. Add the 2 tablespoons lemongrass, the 2 garlic cloves, and the 3 chili peppers, and cook for 2 minutes more.

3 With a slotted spoon, transfer the tofu to a warmed dish. Add the coconut milk and water to the pan and simmer over low heat for 30 minutes. Add the sweet potatoes and simmer for 20 minutes more. Return the tofu to the pan and add the onion. Simmer for 5 minutes.

4 Arrange the curry over the cooked rice sticks and serve hot.

TAKE A CHANCE:

● Serve over cooked rice or soba noodles instead of the rice sticks.

● Add more Thai chili peppers if you dare! If they are not available, use red or green jalapeño or serrano peppers.

● Use 1½ teaspoons grated lemon zest instead of the lemongrass.

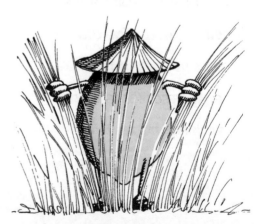

Lemon-Kissed Soy Burgers

*S*eal your veggie burger with the kiss of lemon. *Delicious!*

grated zest and juice of 1 medium lemon

1 large garlic clove, finely minced

1 teaspoon chopped fresh sage, or ½ teaspoon dried

1 teaspoon chopped fresh oregano, or ½ teaspoon dried

2 cups cooked soybeans, mashed, or your favorite veggie burger mix

1 large egg

1 tablespoon Worcestershire sauce

½ tablespoon freshly ground black pepper

SERVES: 4　PREPARATION TIME: 20 MINUTES

1 Combine all of the ingredients, mixing thoroughly. Shape the mixture into 4 large patties.

2 Place the patties on a hot barbecue grill and cook for 5 minutes on each side, turning carefully with a spatula. Or, cook the patties indoors over an electric grill for 5 minutes on each side, or place in a large skillet with 2 tablespoons Mock Lemon Butter (see page 235), melted, and sauté over medium high heat until nicely browned, about 3 to 4 minutes on each side. Serve with lettuce and tomato on whole wheat buns.

TAKE A CHANCE:

- Add ½ teaspoon cayenne pepper or chili powder.
- Make stuffed burgers. Shape 8 thin patties and place mushrooms, chopped onion, or tofu cheese in the middle of 4. Top with the other 4 and seal the edges by pinching them together. Adjust the cooking time so that the cheese melts thoroughly.
- Use lemon thyme instead of the zest.

Lemonaid

Because of its acid content, lemon juice is a terrific marinade for chicken.

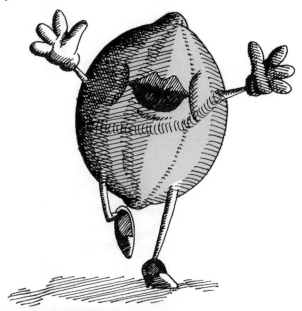

Surprise Packages

Who says you can't have a surprise at the dinner table? Let everyone open their packet and find a delicious veggie burger with all the fixings.

4 uncooked Lemon-Kissed Soy Burgers (see page 127), or your favorite veggie burgers

1 large tomato, thinly sliced

½ medium onion, cut into thin rings

½ teaspoon dried oregano

¼ teaspoon freshly ground black pepper

½ medium lemon, thinly sliced

1 tablespoon chopped fresh parsley

SERVES: 4   PREPARATION TIME: 45 MINUTES

1 Arrange 4 sheets of aluminum foil, each approximately 12-x-12-inches, on the counter.

2 Place one burger on each sheet of aluminum. Arrange tomato slices and onion rings on the top of each burger. Add oregano and pepper to each packet and arrange lemon slices on top. Sprinkle the chopped parsley over the lemon slices.

3 Wrap each burger in its foil, crimping the edges tightly to seal. Place the sealed packets on a cookie sheet and bake in a 350°F oven for 25 minutes, or until the burgers are heated all the way through.

4 Remove the packets from the oven and serve immediately with Lemon Bulgur Pilaf (see page 130).

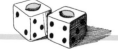

TAKE A CHANCE:

- Add sliced mushrooms.
- Cook on the grill (take them along on your next camping trip).
- Add slices of feta cheese.
- Add fresh basil.

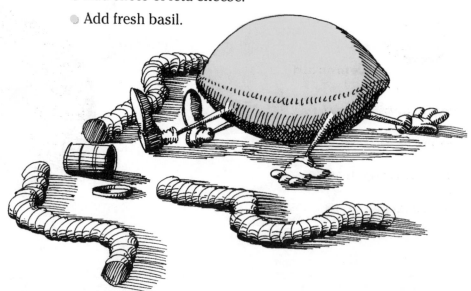

Unmeatloaf With Lemon Sauce

*L*oaf—meat or meatless—
has been on the losing side
*of many jokes over the years.
Well, the joke is now on anyone
who serves this type of dish
without something lemony.*

Loaf

3 tablespoons Lemon
Vegetable Broth (see page 86)

½ cup minced onion

grated zest of 1 medium
lemon

2 small garlic cloves, minced

1 large tomato, seeded and
minced

2 cups cooked and puréed
soybeans

1½ cups cooked bulgur
wheat

1 large egg

½ teaspoon dried sage

½ teaspoon dried thyme

2 tablespoons minced fresh
parsley

Sauce

1½ cups Lemon Vegetable
Broth (see page 86)

¼ cup minced onion

grated zest and juice of 1
medium lemon

1 small garlic clove, minced

1 tablespoon arrowroot

1 large egg

¼ teaspoon freshly ground
black pepper

SERVES: 4   PREPARATION TIME: 1½ HOURS

1 To make the loaf, heat the 3 tablespoons of broth in a large skillet and sauté the ½ cup minced onion for 2 minutes. Add the lemon zest, 2 minced garlic cloves, and tomato, and sauté for 1 minute. Remove the skillet from the heat, add the remaining loaf ingredients except the parsley, and mix well.

2 Shape the mixture into a loaf, pat into a greased 9-x-5-inch loaf pan, and bake in a 350°F oven for 1 hour.

3 To make the sauce, heat 2 tablespoons of the broth in a small saucepan and sauté the ¼ cup minced onion for 2 minutes. Add the lemon zest and 1 minced garlic clove, and sauté for another minute.

4 Add the arrowroot and stir until the liquid is absorbed. Slowly add the remaining broth, stirring constantly and removing any lumps that form. Bring the sauce to a boil, still stirring constantly until the sauce thickens. Add the lemon juice and 1 egg, and stir for 1 minute more. Add the pepper and stir.

5 Remove the loaf from the oven. Remove from the pan and let stand for 5 minutes. Cut into slices and ladle sauce on top. Garnish with parsley and serve with steamed vegetables.

TAKE A CHANCE:

- Serve with Fresh Lemony Salsa (see page 59).
- Add 6 drops hot sauce to the Lemon Sauce.
- Plump up a dried black mushroom in hot water, sliver it, and add to the loaf.
- Add 1 teaspoon shoyu or tamari sauce.

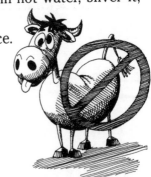

Lemon Bulgur Pilaf

This pilaf is delicious on its own and excellent with steamed fresh vegetables.

grated zest and juice of 1 medium lemon

2 cups Lemon Vegetable Broth (see page 86)

1 large onion, chopped

1½ cups uncooked bulgur wheat

2 tablespoons pine nuts, toasted

SERVES: 4   PREPARATION TIME: 25 MINUTES

1 Heat the lemon juice and 2 tablespoons of the broth in a small saucepan. Add the onion and sauté for 2 minutes. Add the bulgur and stir for 2 minutes, or until the bulgur absorbs the liquid.

2 Add the remaining broth to the bulgur and bring to a boil over high heat. Reduce the heat to low, cover, and cook for 15 minutes. The bulgur should be tender but still chewy. If necessary, add more broth or some water to the bulgar and continue cooking until done. Stir in the lemon zest.

3 Garnish with the pine nuts and serve with steamed vegetables or Lemon-Showered Vegetable Ragout (see page 187).

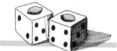

TAKE A CHANCE:

- Add raisins plumped in hot water.
- Add ½ teaspoon chopped fresh basil or rosemary.
- Use rice or barley instead of the bulgur.
- Use walnuts instead of the pine nuts.

Lemonaid

Mix an egg white with a teaspoon of lemon juice for a skin-firming facial mask.

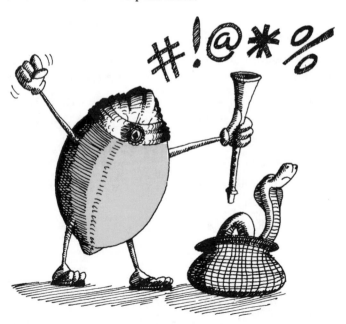

Brown Rice Mexican Style

*S*erve this as a hearty one-
dish meal, or pair it up
with our Citrus Vegetable Fajitas
(see page 115).

2 ripe medium avocados,
peeled, pitted, and sliced

juice of 1 medium lemon

1 tablespoon light sesame
or safflower oil

1 medium onion, coarsely
chopped

1 large garlic clove, minced

1 cup brown rice

$2\frac{1}{2}$ cups water

1 cup corn

1 cup green peas

$\frac{1}{4}$ teaspoon freshly ground
black pepper

Fresh Lemony Salsa
(see page 59)

SERVES: 4   PREPARATION TIME: 1 HOUR

1 In a small bowl, mix the avocado with 1 tablespoon of the lemon juice and set aside.

2 Heat the oil in a medium-sized saucepan and sauté the onion for 2 minutes. Add the garlic and continue sautéing for 1 minute. Add the rice and sauté for another minute.

3 Add the water to the rice mixture and bring to a boil. Reduce the heat to low, cover, and cook for 40 minutes. There should still be some water left in the pan. Add the corn and peas, and continue cooking for 5 minutes, or until the water is absorbed.

4 Stir the remaining lemon juice and the pepper into the rice mixture, garnish with the avocado slices, and serve with the Fresh Lemony Salsa and crisp tortilla chips.

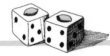

TAKE A CHANCE:

- Sprinkle some grated tofu cheese on top.
- Add 1 diced red or green jalapeño pepper along with the corn and peas.
- Garnish with ¼ cup chopped scallions or cilantro.

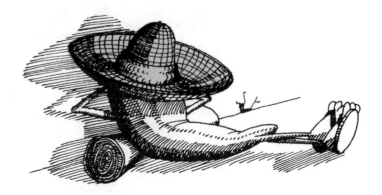

Baked Lemon Rice With Mushrooms and Peas

L iven up those tired every-day rice dishes with a tart bit of lemony goodness.

grated zest and juice of 1 medium lemon

2 teaspoons light sesame or safflower oil

½ cup finely chopped onion

1 cup short-grain brown rice

2 cups water

1 cup green peas

½ pound mushrooms, sliced

⅛ teaspoon freshly ground black pepper

SERVES: 4   PREPARATION TIME: 1¼ HOURS

1 Heat the lemon zest, lemon juice, and oil in a small saucepan over medium heat. Add the onion and sauté for 1 minute. Add the rice and continue cooking for 1 minute. Pour the mixture into a 1½-quart casserole dish, add the water, cover, and bake in a 350°F oven for 50 minutes.

2 Add the peas and mushrooms to the casserole, cover, and continue baking for 10 minutes, or until the rice is tender.

3 Add the pepper, mix well, and serve with Romaine With Olive Oil and Lemon (see page 65).

TAKE A CHANCE:

● Use brown basmati rice instead of the short-grain rice.

● Use Lemon Vegetable Broth (see page 86) instead of the water.

● Omit the lemon zest and add some chopped lemongrass.

● Instead of baking, steam on the stovetop, covered, for 45 minutes.

● Add zucchini slices to the casserole.

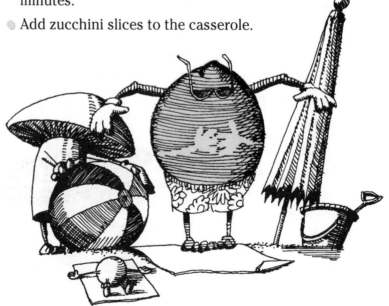

Lemon Risotto With Vegetables

*R*ice picks up a wonderful lemony taste when sautéed with lemon juice.

3¾ cups Lemon Vegetable Broth (see page 86)

½ medium onion, finely chopped

2 large garlic cloves, finely minced

juice of 1 medium lemon

1 cup short-grain brown rice

2 small zucchini, cut in half lengthwise and sliced into ½-inch pieces

2 small crookneck squash, cut in half lengthwise and sliced into ½-inch pieces

1 small red bell pepper, seeded and cut into matchstick-sized pieces

¼ cup snow peas, trimmed

¼ cup finely minced fresh parsley

SERVES: 4   PREPARATION TIME: 1 HOUR

1 In a small saucepan, bring 3½ cups of the Lemon Vegetable Broth to a boil. Lower the heat to a simmer.

2 Heat the remaining broth in a large skillet. Add the onion and sauté over low heat for 1 minute. Add the garlic and continue sautéing for 2 or 3 minutes. Don't let the garlic burn or it will taste bitter. Add the lemon juice and rice to the skillet and stir constantly until the rice absorbs the liquid and is mixed with the onion and garlic, 3 to 5 minutes.

3 Slowly add 1 cup of the warmed broth to the rice and stir constantly until it has been absorbed. Add another ½ cup of the broth and stir until absorbed.

4 Add all the vegetables except the snow peas with another ½ cup of the broth. Continue stirring until the broth is absorbed. Continue adding ½ cup of broth at a time until only ½ cup is left to be added. This will take approximately 20 to 25 minutes.

5 Add the snow peas with the last of the broth and stir until absorbed. The rice will be tender and the vegetables crisp.

6 Sprinkle with the minced parsley and serve.

TAKE A CHANCE:

- Vary the vegetables used. Try mushrooms, broccoli, or asparagus, alone or in any combination.
- Top with grated Parmesan or crumbled feta cheese.
- Sprinkle with chopped walnuts.
- Add chopped fresh basil or oregano just before serving.
- Use cilantro instead of the parsley.

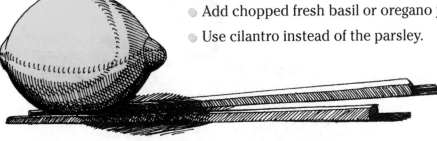

Basmati Rice With Lemongrass

A wonderful change from ordinary rice, basmati is an aromatic rice with a nutty taste. The addition of lemongrass gives it a very subtle lemon flavor.

1 large stalk fresh or dried lemongrass

2 cups brown basmati rice

1 teaspoon light sesame or safflower oil

½ cup finely chopped onion

2 cups water

2 tablespoons chopped fresh cilantro

SERVES: 4   PREPARATION TIME: 1 HOUR

1 If using fresh lemongrass, slice the stalk in half lengthwise. If using dried lemongrass, soak the plant in hot water for 2 hours before cutting, then use only the bottom third of the stalk. Set aside.

2 Place the rice in a colander and rinse under cold running water. Set aside.

3 Heat the oil in a medium-sized saucepan and sauté the onion for 2 minutes. Add the rice and lemongrass, and sauté for another minute. Add the water and bring the rice almost to a boil. Reduce the heat to low, cover, and simmer until the rice is tender and the liquid is absorbed, about 15 minutes. Remove the pan from the heat and let stand for 5 minutes.

4 Discard the lemongrass and fluff the rice with a fork. Garnish with the cilantro and serve with Steamed Vegetable Medley With Lemon and Shoyu (see page 186).

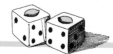

TAKE A CHANCE:

- Garnish with finely minced scallions.
- Use 1½ teaspoons of lemon zest instead of the lemongrass.
- Use chopped shallots instead of the onion.
- Sprinkle with a dash of cayenne pepper before serving.

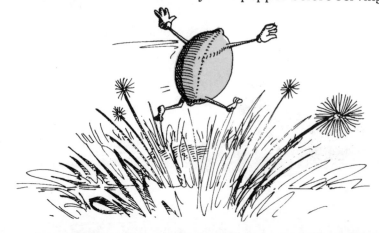

Citrus-Studded Wild Rice

The nutty flavor of the wild rice is complemented by the subtle citrus essence.

2 cups wild rice

6 cups water

2 thin slices of lemon, peeled, sectioned, and coarsely chopped

2 thin slices of orange, peeled, sectioned, and coarsely chopped

SERVES: 4   PREPARATION TIME: 1 HOUR

1 Place the rice in a colander and rinse under cold running water. Place the rinsed rice and the 6 cups water in a medium-sized saucepan and bring to a boil over high heat. Lower the heat and cook for 50 minutes, stirring occasionally. Drain.

2 Return the rice to the saucepan and add the chopped citrus. Cover and cook over very low heat for 10 minutes, or until the rice is tender.

3 Toss the rice and serve immediately with Zippy Roasted Vegetables (see Page 185).

TAKE A CHANCE:

- Add 1 tablespoon each of lemon and orange juice to the cooking water.

- Garnish with toasted sliced almonds.

- Substitute this mixture for the stuffing in Tofu With Citrus Stuffing (see page 120).

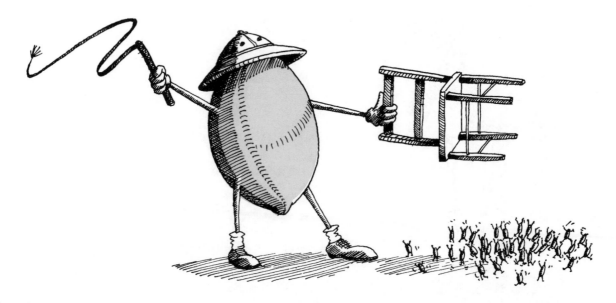

Lemony Couscous

Considered the national dish of Morocco, couscous is finally starting to catch on around the world.

1½ cups water

1 cup couscous

grated zest and juice of 1 medium lemon

SERVES: 4   PREPARATION TIME: 10 MINUTES

1 Bring the water to a boil in a medium-sized saucepan. Add the couscous and lemon zest, and stir. Remove the pan from the heat and cover. Let stand for 5 minutes.

2 Add the lemon juice and fluff the couscous with a fork. Serve with Steamed Vegetable Medley With Lemon and Shoyu (see page 186) or Tofu Stew With Lemons and Olives (see page 124).

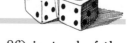

TAKE A CHANCE:

- Use Lemon Vegetable Broth (see page 86) instead of the water and make Couscous Pilaf.

- Mix in a dash of powdered cinnamon or add a cinnamon stick along with the couscous and zest.

- Add ½ teaspoon cayenne pepper.

- Add raisins plumped in hot water or stir in cashews.

- For a more traditional flavor, sprinkle the couscous with 1 tablespoon orange flower or rose water just before serving.

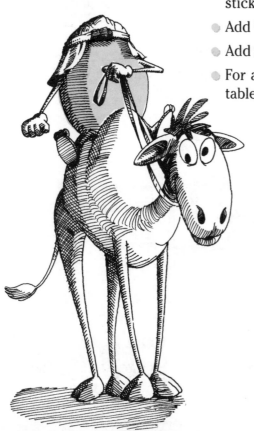

Lemony Lentils, Cabbage, and Potatoes

he lemony taste lingers on your tongue long after this luscious meal is finished.

2 cups cooked lentils

$\frac{1}{2}$ cup whole wheat bread crumbs

$\frac{1}{2}$ cup chopped walnuts

1 large egg

$\frac{1}{4}$ teaspoon freshly ground black pepper

2 teaspoons light sesame or safflower oil

1 large onion, cut into rings

2 large garlic cloves, minced

2 tablespoons arrowroot

2 cups Lemon Vegetable Broth (see page 86)

1 medium head cabbage, cored and quartered

4 large potatoes, quartered

juice of 1 medium lemon

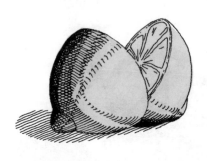

SERVES: 4   PREPARATION TIME: 35 MINUTES

1 Mix the lentils, bread crumbs, walnuts, egg, and pepper together in a large bowl. Shape the mixture into 4 patties.

2 Heat the oil in a deep skillet. Add the patties and brown evenly. Remove the patties from the pan and set aside.

3 Place the onions in the skillet and sauté for 2 minutes. Add the garlic and sauté for another minute. Sprinkle the arrowroot over the mixture and slowly add the broth, stirring constantly so that lumps do not form. Bring the broth to a boil over high heat.

4 Lower the heat to medium and arrange the patties on the bottom of the skillet over the onions. Place one wedge of cabbage on top of each patty. Cover tightly and cook over medium-low heat for 20 minutes, basting the cabbage occasionally with the sauce.

5 While the patties and cabbage are simmering, place the potatoes in a medium-sized saucepan with water to cover and simmer until tender. The potatoes and patties should be done at the same time. Arrange the patties and vegetables on a deep platter and keep warm.

6 Gradually mix the lemon juice into the sauce and cook over low heat for 2 to 3 minutes. Do not boil. Pour the sauce over the patties and vegetables, and serve immediately.

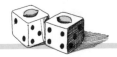

TAKE A CHANCE:

- Mix the lentils with bulgur wheat instead of the walnuts and bread crumbs.

- Use Lemon-Kissed Soy Burgers (see page 127) instead of the lentil patties, omitting the lemon zest.

- Use ½-inch cubes of tofu instead of the lentil patties.

- Cut the potatoes into smaller pieces and cook them in the skillet along with the patties and cabbage. (Be aware that the potatoes can take longer to cook using this method.)

- Sprinkle a dash of paprika or cayenne pepper over each serving.

Vegetable-Nut Logs in Creamy Lemon Sauce

This is a wonderful dish for avowed lemonphiles.

2 cups cooked lentils

1 large egg

½ cup chopped walnuts

½ cup whole grain bread crumbs

¼ teaspoon paprika

¼ teaspoon freshly ground black pepper

1½ cups Lemon Vegetable Broth (see page 86)

3 large shallots, finely minced

½ medium lemon, thinly sliced and then cut into quarters

1 tablespoon arrowroot

juice of 1 medium lemon

½ cup soymilk

¼ cup mashed silken tofu

¼ cup chopped fresh parsley

SERVES: 4   PREPARATION TIME: 45 MINUTES

1 Mix the lentils, egg, walnuts, bread crumbs, paprika, and pepper together in a large bowl. Form the mixture into logs about 3 inches long and 1½ inches wide.

2 Heat 3 tablespoons of the broth in a large skillet. Add the logs and sauté for 3 minutes over medium heat, turning to cook all sides. Remove the logs from the skillet and set aside.

3 Add the shallots and quartered lemon slices to the skillet and sauté for 1 to 2 minutes. Add half of the remaining broth and simmer for 5 minutes. Don't let the shallots or lemon slices burn. Add the arrowroot to the skillet and stir until absorbed. Continue stirring and add the lemon juice and remaining broth. Simmer over low heat for 5 minutes.

4 Add the soymilk and mashed tofu to the skillet and bring to a boil over high heat. Reduce the heat to medium and cook for 1 to 2 minutes more. Return the logs to the skillet and simmer for 10 minutes over low heat, or until the logs are warmed through.

5 Place the logs on a serving platter and pour the sauce on top. Sprinkle with the chopped parsley and serve with Tangy Minted Peas (see page 188) and The Perfect Caesar Salad (see page 66).

TAKE A CHANCE:

● Add chopped fresh sage or thyme or a twig of fresh rosemary to the skillet when you return the logs for heating.

● Use scallions instead of the shallots.

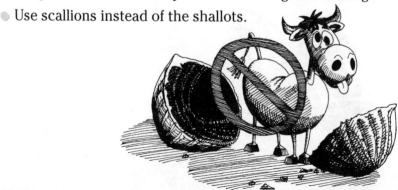

Lemony Vegetable Stir-Fry

This delicious stir-fry is ready in almost no time at all.

6 tablespoons Lemon Vegetable Broth (see page 86)

2 large garlic cloves, slivered

8 ounces fresh spinach, torn into pieces

½ medium lemon, thinly sliced

8 ounces mushrooms, sliced

1 small zucchini, cut into ½-inch slices

1 small crookneck squash, cut into ½-inch slices

1 medium carrot, peeled and cut into matchstick-sized pieces

1 cup broccoli florets

¼ cup snow peas, trimmed

1 tablespoon dried oregano

1 teaspoon dried thyme

¼ teaspoon freshly ground black pepper

grated zest and juice of 1 medium lemon

SERVES: 4   PREPARATION TIME: 30 MINUTES

1 Heat 2 tablespoons of the broth in a large skillet and sauté the garlic for 1 minute. Add the spinach and sauté for 2 minutes, or just until the leaves are wilted. Remove the spinach from the skillet and keep warm in a large dish.

2 Add an additional 2 tablespoons of the broth plus the lemon slices, mushrooms, zucchini, and squash to the skillet and sauté for 2 to 3 minutes. Transfer the vegetables to the dish with the spinach.

3 Add the remaining broth plus the carrots and broccoli to the skillet and sauté for 3 to 4 minutes.

4 Return the cooked vegetables to the skillet and add the snow peas, oregano, thyme, and pepper. Cook over medium heat for 2 to 3 minutes, stirring constantly. The vegetables should still be very crisp. Add the lemon juice and stir well.

5 Transfer the vegetables to a large serving dish. Garnish with the lemon zest and serve over rice or couscous.

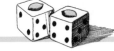

TAKE A CHANCE:

● Sprinkle with sesame seeds or walnuts before serving.

● Use green beans instead of the snow peas.

● Add bean sprouts.

● Add a touch of fire by cooking 2 or 3 dried red peppers along with the garlic.

● Add 8 ounces firm tofu, cut into ½-inch cubes and sauteéd until golden brown.

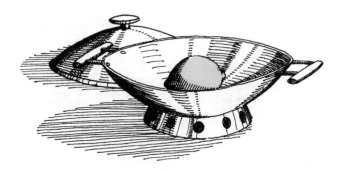

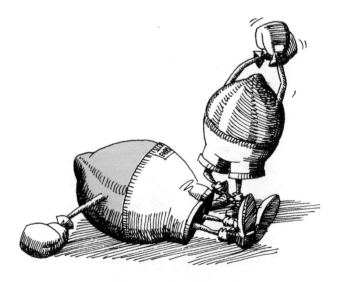

Chapter 7

Dinner Fare—
Tangy Chicken and Fish Entrées

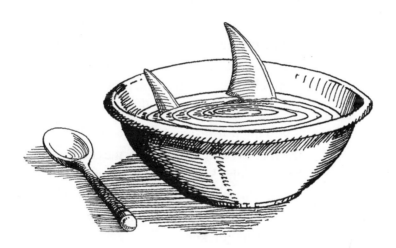

As more people opt for healthier lifestyles, the consumption of low-fat, low-calorie poultry and seafood continues to rise. Chicken and fish easily absorb seasonings and can be used as the basis for many imaginative dishes. Lemon lovers enjoy these foods because their delicate flavors are wonderfully enhanced by citrus. The recipes in this chapter are a few of our favorite creations.

Chicken and fish are not *always* healthy alternatives, however. The following information is therefore presented to help you select the freshest and best-tasting poultry and seafood available. You will also learn how to store and prepare these foods.

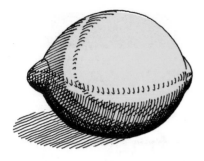

Use Free-Range Chickens

The poultry industry has answered the public's demand for healthier meats with the breeding of free-range chickens and turkeys. Once very rare, free-range chickens are now regularly available in health food stores, co-ops, and specialty and gourmet stores, as well as in many meat markets, supermarkets, and grocery stores.

The most healthful and flavorful free-range chickens were fed organic grains and were not given any growth hormones. The quality of the feed and lack of hormones should be noted on the butcher's sign or on the label. If you are not sure, ask the butcher before you buy the chicken. Try to buy fresh chicken and to cook it on the day of purchase. Freezing will change the flavor a little.

If you must freeze chicken, seal it in an airtight plastic bag or freezer wrap. Be sure to mark the date on the package because chicken should be frozen only up to three months. Thaw the chicken in the refrigerator. A 3½-pound whole chicken will take about a day to thaw. Never refreeze uncooked chicken.

Fresh chicken can be kept in the refrigerator for up to two days wrapped loosely in aluminum foil. Always remove chicken from the store wrapper immediately and wash it thoroughly in cold water with a little lemon juice.

When buying chicken, allow eight ounces per serving if the bones have been removed, or twelve to sixteen ounces per serving if you're using the whole chicken or chicken parts. We also recommend removing the skin before cooking. You see, it is the skin of the chicken that contains most of the fat; the chicken meat alone is relatively low in fat. (By the way, you may want to try free-range turkey in place of chicken for some of the recipes. The flavor is a bit stronger, but the results are equally satisfying.)

Because free-range chickens and turkeys are fed in a more natural way, they take almost twice the time to mature as do mass-produced chickens and turkeys, which are force-fed and often given growth hormones. While the added time to mature means that the price per pound is anywhere from thirty to fifty cents higher for free-range chickens, these chickens are well worth the cost. Organically-fed free-range chickens are not only healthier, but they taste better, too.

Buy the Freshest Fish

When buying fish for dinner, always choose the freshest available. Modern transportation methods have made it much easier for the consumer to purchase fresh fish almost anywhere in the country. At the least, buy fish that has been fresh-frozen without chemical additives or extra processing.

The most important step you can take to find fresh fish is to find a good fish store or market. The fish must be carefully handled and kept properly chilled during transport from boat to market. Quality fish markets know how to handle fish properly, but those stores that sell low volumes or only occasionally handle fresh fish will not always have the knowledge or storage facilities needed to keep fish in optimum condition. If you don't trust the handler, don't buy the fish.

Fish fillets and steaks should never have brown spots or yellow edges. The flesh should be firm rather than spongy, and whole fish should be plump and have clear eyes that bulge slightly. If you're unsure about a fish, ask to smell it. If it smells "fishy," it's not fresh. Fresh fish should give off only a hint of the ocean or stream.

To keep fish at its freshest, dip it in a pan of cool water that has had a teaspoon of lemon juice added. Carefully pat it dry with paper toweling. Unskinned whole fish that has been gutted can be placed directly on ice in a large dish on the bot-

Lemonaid

Removing the skin, the fatty parts at the cavity opening, and the fat from the chicken parts can reduce fat up to 30 percent.

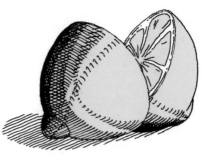

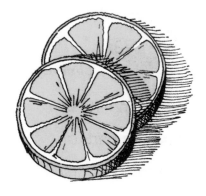

tom shelf of the refrigerator. Fish steaks and fillets should be wrapped in plastic wrap before being put on ice on the bottom refrigerator shelf. Handled correctly, fresh fish can be kept in the refrigerator for up to four days.

When defrosting fresh-frozen fillets, never let them sit submerged in water, as they will become soggy. If you need to quickly defrost frozen fish or chicken, first place it in a resealable plastic bag. Press out the air, seal the bag tightly, and drop it into a large pot of cool water. Do not use hot water, as it will begin the cooking process on the outside too early, altering the taste. The difference in temperature between the frozen fish and the cool water will still be great enough to speed along the defrosting.

How much fish should you prepare? A good rule of thumb is to allow six to eight ounces per serving.

Always Wash Chicken and Fish Before Cooking

To avoid the introduction of salmonella bacteria and other contaminants that can taint your dishes, always rinse your chicken or fish with cool water before cooking. A small amount of lemon juice added to the rinse will also help to keep these foods fresh. In many recipes, the fish or chicken should be patted dry with paper toweling before further preparation. If this is required, it is noted in our instructions. If drying is not specified, leave the fish or chicken wet, but not dripping, as you complete the recipe steps. In all cases, chicken and fish must be thoroughly cooked to be truly safe.

The safe handling of fish and chicken during food preparation extends to your kitchen utensils as well. After raw chicken or fish is removed from a cutting board or dish, the board or dish must be washed thoroughly before other food is placed on or in it. Also, be sure to rinse the knives or other tools used in the preparation of the chicken or fish.

Chicken Stew With Preserved Lemon

This satisfying dinner is made even more enjoyable with the addition of a little lemon.

1 tablespoon shoyu or tamari sauce

2 teaspoons canola oil

1 free-range chicken (4 pounds), skinned and cut into pieces

1 large onion, chopped

2 cups Lemon Vegetable Broth (see page 86)

$1\frac{1}{2}$ teaspoons arrowroot

$\frac{1}{4}$ Moroccan Preserved Lemon (see page 246)

$\frac{1}{2}$ teaspoon chopped fresh dill

SERVES: 4   PREPARATION TIME: $1\frac{1}{4}$ HOURS

1 Heat the shoyu or tamari sauce and the oil in a large skillet over medium heat. Add the chicken and brown on both sides. Transfer the chicken to a plate.

2 Add the onion to the skillet and sauté for 2 minutes.

3 Return the chicken to the skillet and add as much of the broth as needed to cover the chicken. Cover the skillet and simmer for 50 minutes.

4 In a small bowl, dissolve the arrowroot in 2 tablespoons of the pan liquid. Return the liquid to the skillet and stir well. Continue simmering the chicken until the pan liquid thickens, about 5 minutes.

5 Rinse the preserved lemon under cold water. Cut away the fruit and discard. Finely mince the peel, add to the skillet and mix well.

6 Stir in the dill. Serve over Basmati Rice With Lemongrass (see page 134).

TAKE A CHANCE:

- Add the finely chopped fruit of the Moroccan Preserved Lemon to the stew for more lemon tang.

- Use broth from Chicken Noodle Soup With a Drop of Lemon (see page 103) instead of the Lemon Vegetable Broth.

- Use the grated zest of 1 lemon instead of the Moroccan Preserved Lemon.

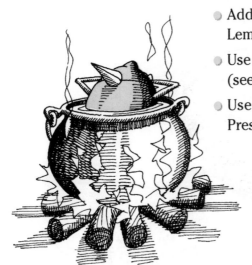

Lemon Basil Chicken Sauté

This recipe is fast, good, and lemony. It is sure to satisfy.

2 tablespoons shoyu or tamari sauce

2 teaspoons lime juice

4 free-range chicken breasts, skinned, boned, and cut into ½-inch cubes

2 tablespoons canola oil

1 tablespoon white wine vinegar

2 large shallots, thinly sliced

2 medium serrano chili peppers, seeded and finely chopped

½ cup coarsely chopped lemon basil

SERVES: 4 PREPARATION TIME: 20 MINUTES

1 Combine 1 tablespoon of the shoyu or tamari sauce and all of the lime juice in a large bowl and toss with the chicken. Set aside.

2 Heat the oil, vinegar, and remaining shoyu or tamari sauce in a large skillet over high heat. Add the shallots and chilies, and sauté for 1 minute.

3 Add the chicken and marinade, and sauté over high heat for 3 minutes, or until the chicken is cooked, stirring constantly. Add the lemon basil and sauté for 1 minute more. Serve with Basmati Rice With Lemongrass (see page 134) and Saucy Lemon Asparagus Bundles (see page 175).

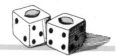

TAKE A CHANCE:

● Omit the lemon basil. Instead, add 1 tablespoon chopped lemongrass to the skillet and garnish with regular basil.

● Add 1 tablespoon grated lemon zest to the skillet.

● Use jalapeño peppers or crushed red pepper instead of the serrano chili peppers.

● Sprinkle with 2 tablespoons chopped peanuts.

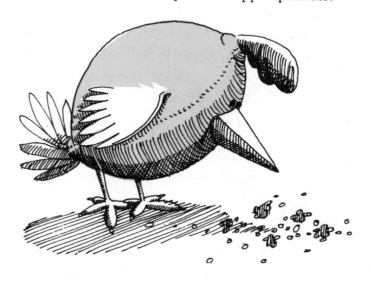

Chicken and Pasta With Tomato Lemon Basil Sauce

This tasty pasta is enhanced by the piquant flavor of lemon basil.

4 free-range chicken breasts, skinned and boned

grated zest and juice of 1 medium lemon

¼ teaspoon freshly ground black pepper

1 tablespoon extra virgin olive oil

2 large garlic cloves, chopped

4 large tomatoes, diced

1 cup Lemon Vegetable Broth (see page 86)

1 pound whole grain tubular pasta such as penne, rigatoni, or mostaccioli

3 cups fresh lemon basil, cut into strips

2 tablespoons freshly grated Parmesan cheese

SERVES: 4   PREPARATION TIME: 45 MINUTES

1 In a medium-sized bowl, toss the chicken with the lemon juice and pepper. Set aside for 10 minutes.

2 Heat the oil in a large skillet and sauté the garlic for 1 minute over medium heat. Add the tomato and sauté for another minute. Add the broth and cook over low heat for 10 to 15 minutes, stirring occasionally.

3 Place the chicken on a broiler pan coated with nonstick cooking spray and broil for 1½ minutes on each side. The chicken will not be completely cooked. Remove it from the pan and cut into ½-inch bite-sized strips.

4 Fill a large pot with water and bring to a full boil. Add the pasta and cook until al dente, about 10 to 12 minutes. Drain, reserving ¼ cup of the cooking water.

5 Add the chicken, lemon zest, and lemon basil to the tomato mixture and cook for 2 minutes, or until the chicken is done.

6 In a large bowl, combine the pasta with the tomato mixture. If the pasta seems too dry, add some of the reserved cooking water or additional broth. Serve immediately with the grated cheese on the side.

TAKE A CHANCE:

- Cook the chicken on the barbecue.
- Cut the chicken into strips before cooking and sauté for 2 minutes in the olive oil. Transfer the chicken to a plate, add the garlic to the skillet, and follow the recipe as stated.
- Use fresh lemon mint or regular basil instead of the lemon basil.
- Add ¼ teaspoon crushed red pepper to the tomato mixture.
- Use tofu-Parmesan instead of the regular Parmesan.
- Use farfalle pasta (bow ties) instead of the tubular pasta.
- Use shrimp instead of the chicken.

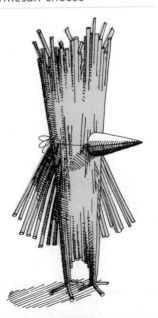

Lemon Chicken and Broccoli Stir-Fry

Serve this quick citrus stir-fry with wild rice for a satisfying twist.

4 free-range chicken breasts, skinned, boned, and cut into $\frac{1}{2}$-inch cubes

juice of 1 medium lemon

$\frac{1}{4}$ teaspoon freshly grated ginger

1 tablespoon shoyu or tamari sauce

$\frac{1}{4}$ teaspoon freshly ground black pepper

1 teaspoon hot chili pepper oil

2 scallions, coarsely chopped

6 thin lemon slices, cut into quarters

$\frac{1}{2}$ cup Lemon Vegetable Broth (see page 86)

2 cups broccoli florets

$\frac{1}{2}$ cup bean sprouts

2 tablespoons chopped peanuts

SERVES: 4   PREPARATION TIME: 25 MINUTES

1 In a medium-sized bowl, toss the chicken with the lemon juice, ginger, shoyu or tamari sauce, and pepper. Set aside for 5 minutes.

2 Heat the oil in a large skillet and sauté the chicken and marinade for 2 minutes over medium-high heat. Transfer the chicken to a warm plate.

3 Place the scallion in the skillet and sauté over medium heat for 1 minute. Add the lemon and sauté for another minute.

4 Add the broth and broccoli to the skillet and cook for 3 minutes.

5 Return the chicken to the skillet and add the bean sprouts. Stir-fry for 1 minute, or until the chicken is warmed through.

6 Arrange the stir-fry on a large serving dish, sprinkle with the peanuts, and serve with bowls of rice.

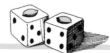

TAKE A CHANCE:

- Omit the ground black pepper and add 6 Szechwan peppercorns—either whole or crushed—to the marinade.
- Use snow peas instead of the bean sprouts.
- Add ½ cup sliced mushrooms along with the broccoli.
- Use light sesame oil instead of the hot chili pepper oil.

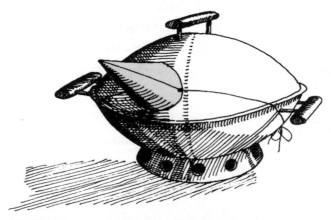

Lemon Sesame Chicken

The sesame seeds add a nutty crunch to this oven-fried chicken, while the yogurt keeps it moist.

1 free-range chicken
(3 pounds), skinned and cut
into pieces

grated zest and juice of 1
medium lemon

1 cup plain nonfat yogurt

½ cup whole wheat bread
crumbs

½ teaspoon dried thyme

½ teaspoon paprika

¼ teaspoon freshly ground
black pepper

¼ cup sesame seeds

SERVES: 4   PREPARATION TIME: 1¼ HOURS

1 Rinse the chicken pieces under cold water and pat dry with paper toweling.

2 In a large bowl, combine the lemon zest, lemon juice, and yogurt, mixing well. Set aside.

3 On a large plate, combine the bread crumbs, seasonings, and sesame seeds. Coat the chicken pieces with the yogurt mixture, then roll in the bread crumbs.

4 Place the coated chicken pieces on an ungreased medium-sized baking pan and bake in a 350°F oven for 1 hour, or until the chicken is cooked through. Serve with Zippy Roasted Vegetables (see page 185) and Baked Potatoes With Almost Sour Cream (see page 171).

TAKE A CHANCE:

● Omit the paprika and add ¼ to ½ teaspoon cayenne pepper instead.

● Use nonfat sour cream instead of the yogurt.

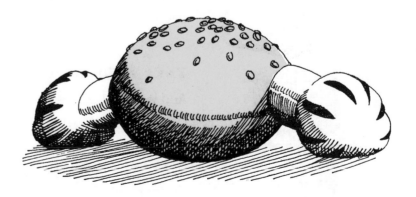

Southwestern Lemon Chicken

A desert delight that melds the "picante" of chilies with the wonderful tang of lemons.

1 free-range chicken (4 pounds), skinned and cut into pieces

3 large dried red chili peppers

$\frac{1}{2}$ cup boiling water

1 tablespoon canola oil

1 medium onion, chopped

4 large jalapeño peppers, seeded and finely chopped

2 large garlic cloves, chopped

grated zest and juice of 1 medium lemon

1 cup Lemon Vegetable Broth (see page 86)

3 large tomatoes, diced

$\frac{1}{4}$ cup minced fresh cilantro

SERVES: 4   PREPARATION TIME: 45 MINUTES

1 Rinse the chicken pieces under cold water and pat dry with paper toweling.

2 Break the red chilies into small pieces, place in a small bowl, and cover with the boiling water. (Wear rubber gloves if the chilies irritate your skin.)

3 Heat the oil in a large skillet and brown the chicken over medium heat for 5 minutes on each side. Transfer the chicken to a warm plate.

4 Add the onion and jalapeños to the skillet and sauté for 2 minutes. Add the garlic, lemon zest, and lemon juice, and sauté for another minute.

5 Turn the heat up to medium-high and add the broth. Bring to a boil and add the tomato. Lower the heat to medium and cook for 5 minutes, stirring occasionally.

6 Place the red chilies and water in a blender or food processor and blend until smooth. Add to the skillet mixture and stir well.

7 Return the chicken to the skillet, cover, and cook for 20 to 25 minutes, or until the chicken is done.

8 Arrange the chicken on a serving platter, garnish with the cilantro, and serve with Brown Rice Mexican Style (see page 131).

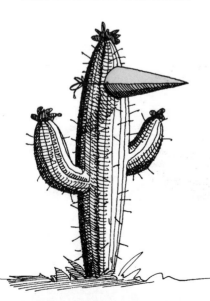

TAKE A CHANCE:

• Add ½ cup diced green bell pepper with the tomato.

• Omit the dried red chilies and use 1 tablespoon crushed red pepper.

• Use ½ cup tomato sauce instead of the fresh tomatoes.

• Use hot chili pepper oil instead of the canola oil.

• Garnish with diced avocado.

Raspberry Lemon Chicken

The tang from the lemon and raspberry vinegar is sure to awaken your taste buds.

1 free-range chicken (3 pounds), skinned and cut into pieces

1 tablespoon canola or light sesame oil

$\frac{1}{2}$ medium lemon, thinly sliced, seeded, and quartered

$\frac{1}{2}$ medium onion, cut lengthwise into $\frac{1}{8}$-inch slices

$\frac{1}{8}$ teaspoon freshly ground black pepper

1 cup Lemon Vegetable Broth (see page 86)

$\frac{1}{4}$ cup raspberry vinegar

$\frac{1}{4}$ cup raspberries, hulled

12 fresh mint leaves

SERVES: 4   PREPARATION TIME: 45 MINUTES

1 Rinse the chicken pieces under cold water and pat dry with paper toweling.

2 Heat the oil in a large skillet and brown the chicken over medium heat for about 5 minutes on each side. Transfer the chicken to a plate.

3 Add the lemon, onion, and pepper to the skillet and sauté for 2 minutes. Add the broth and vinegar, and bring the mixture to a boil over high heat. Lower the heat to medium and return the chicken to the skillet. Cover and cook for 20 to 25 minutes, or until the chicken is tender. Transfer the chicken to a warm plate.

4 Bring the pan liquid to a boil over high heat, stirring constantly for 2 minutes. Spoon the reduced pan liquid along with the lemon and onion over the chicken and garnish with the raspberries and mint. Serve with Parsley Potatoes With Mock Lemon Butter (see page 170) and Luscious Brussels Sprouts (see page 181).

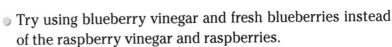

TAKE A CHANCE:

○ Try using blueberry vinegar and fresh blueberries instead of the raspberry vinegar and raspberries.

○ Garnish with toasted almonds.

○ Omit the lemon slices and add the grated zest and juice of 1 medium lemon to the sauté mixture.

○ Use slices of Moroccan Preserved Lemons (see page 246) instead of the fresh lemons.

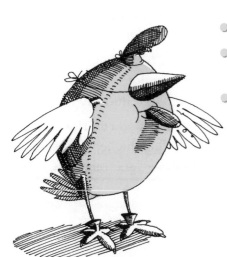

Roasted Citrus Chicken

Moist and tender, with a background of citrus goodness, this is chicken at its Sunday best. Bake with the skin on for a juicier bird, then remove the skin before carving to reduce the fat.

1 whole free-range chicken (4 pounds), trimmed of excess fat

grated zest and juice of 1 medium lemon

grated zest and juice of 1 large orange

$\frac{1}{2}$ teaspoon paprika

$\frac{1}{2}$ teaspoon freshly ground black pepper

1 large shallot, sliced

$1\frac{1}{4}$ cups Lemon Vegetable Broth (see page 86)

SERVES: 4   PREPARATION TIME: $5\frac{1}{4}$ HOURS

1 Rinse the chicken under cold water and pat dry with paper toweling. Place it in a medium-sized roasting pan that has been sprayed with nonstick cooking spray.

2 Mix the lemon and orange juices in a small bowl and pour over the chicken. Leave the juice mixture in the bottom of the roasting pan.

3 Mix the lemon and orange zest together in a small bowl. Rub the inside of the chicken with half of the mixture, leaving the zest in the cavity.

4 Mix the remaining zest with the paprika and pepper, and spread it over the outside of the chicken, using your fingers. Cover the chicken and refrigerate for 4 hours, occasionally spooning the juice over the chicken while marinating.

5 Remove the chicken from the refrigerator. In a small skillet, sauté the shallot in the broth until the broth is very hot, about 2 minutes. Pour the broth into the cavity of the chicken.

6 Bake the chicken, uncovered, in a 350°F oven for $1\frac{1}{4}$ hours, basting occasionally with the pan liquid. You will know the chicken is done when the juices in the thigh run clean after you pierce the thigh with a fork. Transfer the chicken to a warm plate and cover with foil.

7 Pour the remaining pan liquid into a large measuring cup and spoon off any grease. Pour the liquid into a small saucepan and simmer for 10 minutes to reduce by half.

8 Remove the skin from the chicken and carve the meat. Spoon the reduced pan liquid over the chicken and serve with Lemon Lover's Mashed Potatoes (see page 172) or brown rice.

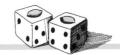

TAKE A CHANCE:

- Omit the grated zest from the cavity mixture and instead use 2 tablespoons lemon basil.

- Try adding ¼ teaspoon each ground sage and thyme to the zest marinade.

- Use Gremolata (see page 228) instead of the citrus zest to stuff and marinate the chicken.

- Use 2 whole pearl onions instead of the shallot.

- Instead of roasting the chicken, bake it in a covered clay pot. It will cook in half the time. Don't open the pot or baste during cooking. When done, the juicy chicken will fall apart without carving.

Lemonaid

Pulse equal parts of dried lemon zest and dried orange zest in a blender until the mixture turns into a fine powder. Apply it liberally as a natural deodorant.

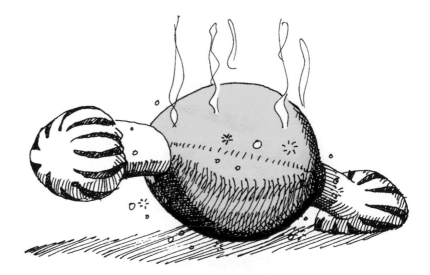

Barbecued Lemon Chicken

There's nothing better for a backyard barbecue than chicken grilled with a luscious lemon sauce. Make sure you have plenty of napkins or warm, damp towels on hand for after-dinner cleanup. Serve with ears of Grilled Herbed Corn on the Cob (see page 179) for summer-time fireworks!

1 free-range chicken
(4 pounds), skinned and
cut into pieces

juice of 1 medium lemon

$\frac{1}{2}$ teaspoon dried oregano

$\frac{1}{2}$ teaspoon dried sage

$\frac{1}{2}$ teaspoon freshly ground
black pepper

2 cups Zesty Barbecue Sauce
(see page 232)

SERVES: 4   PREPARATION TIME: 1$\frac{1}{2}$ HOURS

1 Rinse the chicken pieces under cold water and pat dry with paper toweling.

2 Place the chicken pieces in a single layer on a large platter and drizzle with the lemon juice. Sprinkle the oregano, sage, and pepper over the chicken. Cover and refrigerate for 1 hour, turning the pieces over in the lemon marinade at least once.

3 Grill the chicken over medium heat for 30 minutes, or until almost done. Spread the barbecue sauce on both sides and grill for a final 5 minutes, turning frequently.

4 Place the grilled chicken on a serving platter, pour the remaining barbecue sauce over the chicken, and serve.

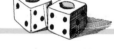

TAKE A CHANCE:

● Add 1 teaspoon chili powder or cayenne pepper to the marinade for a little more fire.

● Omit the barbecue sauce. Instead, marinate and grill the chicken as recommended, but serve with Fresh Lemony Salsa (see page 59).

● Roast the chicken instead of barbecuing it and pour the barbecue sauce over the chicken during the last ten minutes of roasting.

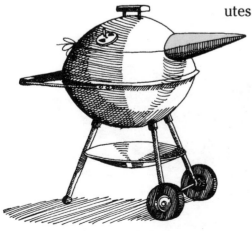

Marinated Swordfish Kabobs

This firm, mild saltwater fish is wonderful grilled, and it loves lemons as much as we do. Marinating helps the fish stay moist during grilling.

Marinade

grated zest and juice of 1 medium lemon

1 large garlic clove, crushed

1 teaspoon dried thyme

$\frac{1}{2}$ teaspoon paprika

$\frac{1}{8}$ teaspoon freshly ground black pepper

2 tablespoons canola or other light oil

Kabobs

$1\frac{1}{2}$ pounds thick swordfish steaks, cut into 2-inch pieces

12 cherry tomatoes

1 small onion, cut into wedges

1 medium green bell pepper, seeded and cut into 1-inch slices

1 medium lemon, cut into wedges

SERVES: 4   PREPARATION TIME: $2\frac{1}{2}$ HOURS

1 To make the marinade, combine all the marinade ingredients in a large bowl and let sit at room temperature for 10 to 20 minutes.

2 Add the fish and vegetables to the marinade, cover, and refrigerate for 2 hours.

3 Alternating the ingredients, thread the fish, tomatoes, onion, and green pepper on metal skewers, or on long bamboo skewers that have been soaked in water for 20 minutes.

4 Coat the barbecue or electric grill with nonstick cooking spray and cook the kabobs over medium heat for 4 to 5 minutes on each side. Baste or brush the kabobs with any remaining marinade as you turn them.

5 Transfer the kabobs to a warm plate and serve with Citrus-Studded Wild Rice (see page 135) and the lemon wedges on the side.

TAKE A CHANCE:

- Add ½ teaspoon chopped fresh dill to the marinade.
- Add mushrooms or zucchini to the kabobs.
- Use tuna steaks instead of the swordfish.

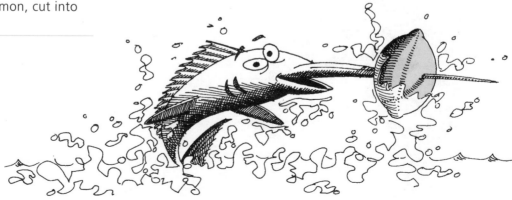

Sassy Orange Roughy

Quick, easy, and nutritious, this dish fits in perfectly with today's healthy lifestyle. The delicate taste of the orange roughy is made sassy with some citrus sunshine.

4 orange roughy fillets (6 to 8 ounces each)

grated zest and juice of 1 medium lemon

⅛ teaspoon freshly ground black pepper

grated zest of 1 medium orange

1 teaspoon grated grapefruit zest

SERVES: 4   PREPARATION TIME: 15 MINUTES

1 Place the fish fillets on a large plate and drizzle with the lemon juice. Turn the fish over so that the lemon juice covers both sides.

2 Place the fish on a broiling pan coated with nonstick cooking spray and sprinkle with the pepper. Broil the fish 5 minutes for each ½-inch of thickness. The fish is done when it flakes easily with a fork and its flesh is opaque white. It is not necessary to turn the fish over during broiling, but you can if you like drier fish or if the fillets are thick.

3 Arrange the fillets on a serving plate and garnish with the lemon, orange, and grapefruit zest. Serve with Baked Lemon Rice With Mushrooms and Peas (see page 132).

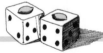

TAKE A CHANCE:

● Use lemon sole or flounder instead of the orange roughy.

● Omit the orange and grapefruit zest and use the zest of 2 medium lemons instead.

● Omit the zest and garnish with chopped lemon mint.

● Pan-fry the fish in a skillet in 2 teaspoons soy butter.

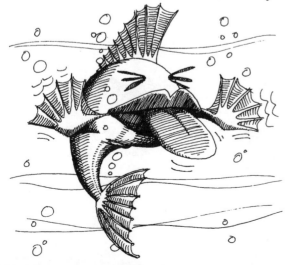

Lemon Shrimp on a Stick

Throw some shrimp on the barbie, and don't forget the lemon!

grated zest and juice of 2 medium lemons

3 tablespoons shoyu or tamari sauce

2 tablespoons extra virgin olive oil

½ teaspoon dried oregano

¼ teaspoon freshly ground black pepper

1 pound medium shrimp, shelled and deveined

1 medium green bell pepper, seeded and cut into ½-inch squares

8 ounces large mushrooms, stems cut flush with the cap

2 tablespoons chopped fresh parsley

1 medium lemon, cut into wedges

SERVES: 4   PREPARATION TIME: 1½ HOURS

1 In a large bowl, combine the lemon zest, lemon juice, shoyu or tamari sauce, oil, oregano, and black pepper. Add the shrimp and mix well. Cover and marinate in the refrigerator for 1 hour.

2 With a slotted spoon, remove the shrimp from the marinade and transfer to a plate. Add the green pepper and mushrooms to the marinade and coat evenly. Using the slotted spoon, remove the vegetables from the marinade and transfer to a plate.

3 Alternating the ingredients, thread the shrimp, green pepper, and mushrooms on metal skewers, or on long bamboo skewers that have been soaked in water for 20 minutes. Place the skewers on a barbecue grill for 10 minutes, or until the shrimp turn pink. Baste with the remaining marinade and turn occasionally.

4 Arrange the skewers on a serving platter, garnish with the parsley, and serve with the lemon wedges and bowls of rice.

TAKE A CHANCE:

- Marinate the green pepper and mushrooms along with the shrimp.

- Marinate and cook the shrimp with their shells on.

- Use red and yellow bell peppers for a different taste, or add ½-inch squares of onion to the skewers.

- Use chicken or scallops instead of the shrimp.

- Skewer the shrimp and vegetables on large rosemary branches stripped of leaves.

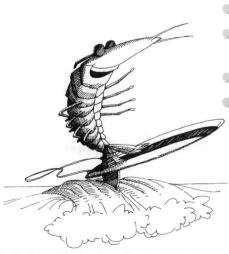

Cod and Zucchini in Lemon Tomato Sauce

S erve this delicious dish over your favorite whole grain pasta for a light and lemony twist on traditional Italian fare.

1 teaspoon extra virgin olive oil

½ medium onion, coarsely chopped

2 large garlic cloves, finely chopped

grated zest and juice of 2 medium lemons

4 large tomatoes, coarsely chopped

4 large zucchini, cut into ½-inch slices

½ teaspoon dried oregano

4 cod fillets
(6 to 8 ounces each)

2 tablespoons finely chopped fresh parsley

SERVES: 4   PREPARATION TIME: 1 HOUR

1 Heat the oil in a large skillet and sauté the onion for 2 minutes over high heat. Add the garlic and half the lemon zest, and sauté for another minute. Add the tomato, reduce the heat to medium-low, and simmer for 20 minutes. Add the zucchini, half of the lemon juice, and the oregano, and cook for another minute.

2 Rinse the fish under cold water and pat dry with paper toweling. Place it in a large baking dish coated with non-stick cooking spray. Drizzle the remaining lemon juice over the fish and cover with the tomato and zucchini sauté.

3 Bake the fish, uncovered, in a 350°F oven for 20 to 25 minutes, or until the fish flakes easily with a fork.

4 Arrange the fish on a serving platter, garnish with the parsley and remaining lemon zest, and serve over pasta.

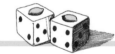

TAKE A CHANCE:

- Use haddock or flounder instead of the cod.
- Add 4 ounces small mushrooms along with the zucchini.
- After cooking the tomatoes for 20 minutes, purée them in a blender. Return them to the skillet and add the zucchini.
- Use rosemary instead of the oregano.

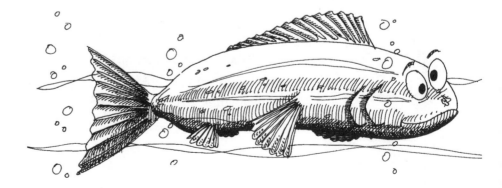

Shark With Lemon Spinach Pesto

The shark becomes a mellow fellow with the addition of this soothing pesto.

4 shark steaks
(8 ounces each)

juice of 1 medium lemon

¼ teaspoon freshly ground
black pepper

1 cup Lemon Spinach Pesto
(see page 109)

1 teaspoon finely chopped
fresh parsley

1 medium lemon, cut into
wedges

Lemonaid

Remove the smell of fish from your fingers by rinsing them in lemon juice or rubbing them with a juiced lemon hull.

SERVES: 4   PREPARATION TIME: 20 MINUTES

1 Rinse the fish under cold water and pat dry with paper toweling. Place the fish on a large plate and drizzle with the lemon juice. Turn the fish over so that the lemon juice covers both sides. Sprinkle with the pepper.

2 Place the fish on a broiler pan coated with nonstick cooking spray and broil for 3 minutes on each side, or until the fish flakes easily with a fork.

3 Arrange the steaks on a serving platter and top each with a dollop of the pesto. Garnish with the parsley and serve with the lemon wedges and Lemon-Showered Vegetable Ragout (see page 187).

TAKE A CHANCE:

○ Use tuna or salmon steaks instead of the shark.

○ Omit the pesto and top the steaks with Fresh Lemony Salsa (see page 59).

○ Instead of broiling the steaks, grill them on the barbecue.

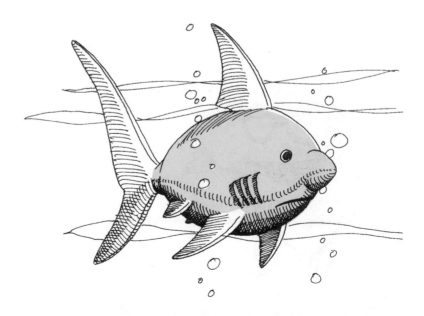

Tuna Poached in Lemon

Poaching makes the fish moist and flaky. The lemony flavor is a tasty bonus.

¾ cup Lemon Vegetable Broth (see page 86)

grated zest and juice of 2 medium lemons

½ cup water

1 thin slice onion, broken into rings

½ teaspoon dried thyme

¼ teaspoon freshly ground black pepper

4 tuna steaks (8 ounces each)

SERVES: 4   PREPARATION TIME: 30 MINUTES

1 Place all the ingredients except the lemon zest and fish in a medium-sized skillet. Cover and bring the mixture to a boil over high heat. Reduce the heat to low and simmer for 5 minutes.

2 Add the fish to the skillet. Cover and simmer for 5 to 10 minutes more, or until the fish flakes easily with a fork. Occasionally spoon the pan liquid over the fish to keep it moist.

3 Transfer the fish to a warm plate and set aside. Remove the onions from the skillet and discard.

4 Bring the pan liquid to a boil and cook for 5 minutes, or until reduced to about ½ to ⅓ cup. Spoon the reduced pan liquid over the fish, garnish with the lemon zest, and serve with Zucchini Lemon Sauté (see page 184).

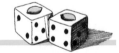

TAKE A CHANCE:

- Use halibut steaks instead of the tuna.

- Add 6 thin slices of lemon to the pan liquid. Discard before serving.

- Omit the onion and add thinly sliced mushrooms and carrots instead. Remove the vegetables from the pan along with the fish and serve.

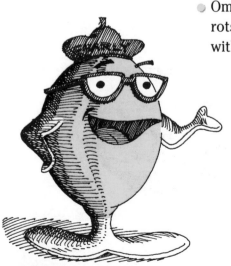

Steamed Lemon Sole

erve this steamed delight over rice to soak up the lemony juices.

grated zest and juice of 1 medium lemon

2 tablespoons shoyu or tamari sauce

1 tablespoon rice vinegar

1 tablespoon canola oil

4 lemon sole fillets
(6 to 8 ounces each)

2 thin slices fresh ginger

2 scallions, cut into quarters

2 tablespoons chopped fresh cilantro

SERVES: 4   PREPARATION TIME: 20 MINUTES

1 Mix the lemon zest, lemon juice, shoyu or tamari sauce, vinegar, and oil in a small bowl.

2 Place the fish in a shallow heat-resistant bowl or plate. Pour the lemon juice mixture over the fish and place the ginger and scallions on top.

3 Cover the fish with a piece of waxed or parchment paper and place the bowl on the rack of a steamer set over boiling water. Cover the steamer and cook the fish for 8 to 10 minutes, or until the fish is flaky but not dry.

4 Transfer the fish to a serving plate and pour the pan liquid over it. Garnish with the cilantro and serve over rice with Lemony Garlic Mushrooms (see page 180).

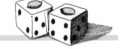

TAKE A CHANCE:

- Add 4 ounces drained firm tofu to the fish while steaming.
- Use sea bass instead of the sole.
- If a steamer is not available, place the fish in a metal colander set over boiling water and heat the sauce in a separate saucepan. Or sauté the fish in a large skillet.
- Use hot chili pepper oil instead of the canola oil.
- Omit the zest and place two slices of lemon over each fish fillet instead.

Lemonaid

The addition of lemon juice to pan liquid helps keep fish firm and white.

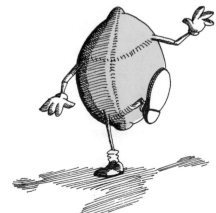

Pasta With Lemon Scallops

The flavor of these tender, succulent scallops is nicely enhanced by the addition of lemon. The pasta helps to soak up the tasty juices.

2 pounds bay scallops

grated zest and juice of 4 medium lemons

$\frac{1}{2}$ teaspoon paprika

$\frac{1}{2}$ teaspoon freshly ground black pepper

6 large garlic cloves, peeled

$\frac{1}{2}$ cup fresh parsley sprigs

1 cup Lemon Vegetable Broth (see page 86)

2 tablespoons chopped fresh oregano, or 2 teaspoons dried

$\frac{1}{2}$ cup extra virgin olive oil

8 ounces thin whole grain pasta such as capellini or vermicelli

SERVES: 4   PREPARATION TIME: 15 MINUTES

1 Place the scallops in a medium-sized bowl and mix with 2 teaspoons of the lemon juice and all of the lemon zest, paprika, and pepper. Set aside.

2 Place the garlic in a blender or food processor and pulse 3 times. Add the parsley and pulse until the garlic and parsley are finely chopped. Add the broth, oregano, and remaining lemon juice, and pulse 3 times.

3 With the motor of the blender or processor running, slowly add the oil and process until completely blended. Turn the machine off.

4 Fill a large pot with water and bring to a full boil. Add the pasta and cook until al dente, 4 to 6 minutes. Drain, reserving ¼ cup of the cooking water, then place in a large serving bowl and keep warm.

5 Place 2 tablespoons of the lemon juice mixture in a small skillet and warm. Add the scallops and sauté over medium heat for 3 to 4 minutes, or until the scallops turn opaque.

6 Add the remaining lemon juice mixture to the pasta and toss. If the pasta seems too dry, add some of the reserved cooking water. Top the pasta with the scallops and serve with Slivers of Lemon and Broccoli (see page 168).

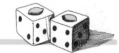

TAKE A CHANCE:

● Add ½ teaspoon grated fresh ginger to the scallops.

● Add ½ teaspoon crushed red pepper to the blender.

● Use cilantro instead of the parsley.

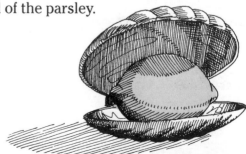

Savory Lemon-Baked Fish Fillets

N o fuss, no muss, no bother, and perfect fish every time.

4 halibut or other white fish fillets (6 to 8 ounces each)

2 teaspoons dried lemon basil

$\frac{1}{4}$ teaspoon freshly ground black pepper

2 medium lemons, thinly sliced

SERVES: 4   PREPARATION TIME: 20 MINUTES

1 Sprinkle the fish fillets with the lemon basil and pepper.

2 Cut 4 sheets of parchment paper or heavy duty aluminum foil, each large enough to fold into a packet around one fish fillet. Distribute half of the lemon slices evenly over the 4 pieces of paper or foil. Place the fish on top of the lemons, and arrange the remaining lemon slices on top of the fish.

3 Fold each piece of paper or foil into a packet around the fish fillets and tightly crimp the edges. Place the packets on a baking sheet or in a large baking pan and bake in a 350°F oven for 8 to 10 minutes, or until the fish turns opaque.

4 Serve the fish still in the packets, with extra lemon slices, Parsley Potatoes With Mock Lemon Butter (see page 170), and melted Mock Lemon Butter (see page 235) on the side.

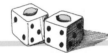

TAKE A CHANCE:

- Add onions, mushrooms, or green bell peppers to each packet.
- Use dill instead of the lemon basil, or sprinkle the fish with paprika or cayenne pepper before baking.
- Place ½ teaspoon unmelted Mock Lemon Butter in each packet before baking.
- Omit the packets. Just place a sheet of foil over the bottom of a baking dish, add the lemons and fish, and bake. Turn the fish once and baste frequently with the pan liquid.
- Cook the packets over low heat on a barbeque grill with the lid down.

Lemonaid

Lemon juice doesn't disguise the taste of fish—it enhances its natural flavor.

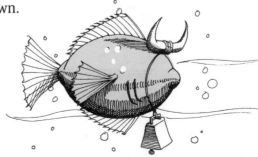

Broiled Lemon Salmon

Broiled salmon is easy to make and tasty, especially when it is topped with Lemony Hollandaise Sauce.

4 salmon steaks
(6 to 8 ounces each)

juice of 1 medium lemon

$\frac{1}{2}$ teaspoon finely chopped fresh dill

$\frac{1}{8}$ teaspoon freshly ground black pepper

$\frac{3}{4}$ cup Lemony Hollandaise Sauce (see page 230)

SERVES: 4   PREPARATION TIME: 40 MINUTES

1 Place the salmon in a shallow dish and drizzle with the lemon juice. Sprinkle the dill and pepper over the fish, cover, and refrigerate for 25 minutes.

2 Arrange the fish on a broiling pan coated with nonstick cooking spray. Broil the steaks for 5 minutes on each side, or until lightly browned. Turn the steaks over again and broil for another 5 minutes on each side, or until the fish is opaque.

3 Transfer the salmon steaks to a large warm platter and drizzle 1 tablespoon of the Lemony Hollandaise Sauce over each one. Serve with Basmati Rice With Lemongrass (see page 134), Tangy Minted Peas (see page 188), and the remaining sauce on the side.

TAKE A CHANCE:

- Use halibut or another type of white fish steaks instead of the salmon.

- Omit the Lemony Hollandaise Sauce and instead serve with Fresh Lemony Salsa (see page 59).

- Use oregano instead of the dill.

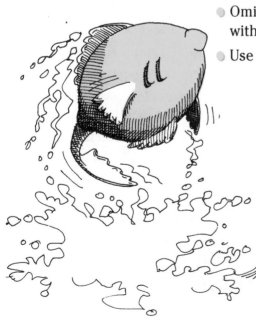

Chapter 8

Veggies on the Side—
A Garden of Lemon Delight

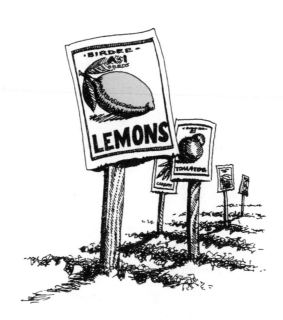

A splash of juice or a dash of zest, and the flavor of even the freshest produce is enhanced. Reach for your trusty lemon instead of butter and taste vegetables prepared as Mother Nature intended. The veggie dishes on the following pages are presented as side dishes, but you may want to serve them in larger portions as the focus of your meal, along with brown rice or another grain as a side dish.

Leeks and Carrots in Lemon Sauce

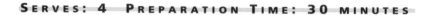

This is a tasty way to get little lemonphiles to eat some of those vegetables they normally won't even allow on their plates.

1¼ cups Lemon Vegetable Broth (see page 86)

2 large garlic cloves, minced

2 cups leeks, white part only, sliced ½-inch thick

2 cups carrots, peeled and sliced ¼-inch thick

1 tablespoon arrowroot

1 tablespoon cold water

1 large egg

juice of 1 medium lemon

¼ teaspoon freshly ground black pepper

2 tablespoons chopped fresh parsley

SERVES: 4   PREPARATION TIME: 30 MINUTES

1 Heat 2 tablespoons of the broth in a large skillet and sauté the garlic and leeks for 3 minutes over medium heat. Add the carrot slices and sauté for 2 more minutes. Add the remaining broth and simmer for 15 minutes.

2 Mix the arrowroot with the cold water in a small bowl. Add 2 tablespoons of the hot broth and stir until blended. Return the broth to the skillet and mix well. Increase the cooking temperature to medium-high and stir constantly until the sauce thickens.

3 Remove the skillet from the heat and stir in the egg, lemon juice, and pepper. Mix thoroughly.

4 Ladle the vegetables and sauce into a large dish, garnish with the parsley, and serve immediately.

Note From a Healthy Lemon:

To make this dish cholesterol-free, replace the egg with an egg substitute.

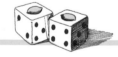

TAKE A CHANCE:

- Garnish with dill or basil instead of the parsley.
- Try using eggplant, green beans, or zucchini instead of the leeks and carrots.
- Add sliced mushrooms to the mixture.

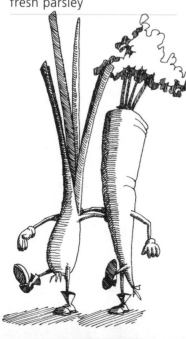

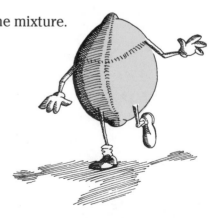

Lemon Carrots Oriental

A touch of oriental mystery and the goodness of lemon make these carrots a special treat.

juice of 1 medium lemon

2 tablespoons shoyu or tamari sauce

1 teaspoon malt syrup

2 teaspoons soy margarine

4 medium carrots, cut into matchstick-sized pieces

4 cilantro sprigs

SERVES: 4   PREPARATION TIME: 15 MINUTES

1 Place the lemon juice, shoyu or tamari sauce, malt syrup, and margarine in a medium-sized saucepan and cook for 1 minute over medium heat. Add the carrots and cook for 5 minutes. The carrots should be very crisp.

2 Place the carrots in a medium-sized dish and pour the sauce from the pan over them. Garnish with the cilantro and serve immediately.

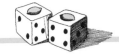

TAKE A CHANCE:

● Add matchstick-sized pieces of zucchini or onion.

● Add 1 small clove crushed garlic.

● Use Lemon Vegetable Broth (see page 86) instead of the soy margarine.

● Omit the lemon juice and add lemon verbena or lemon basil.

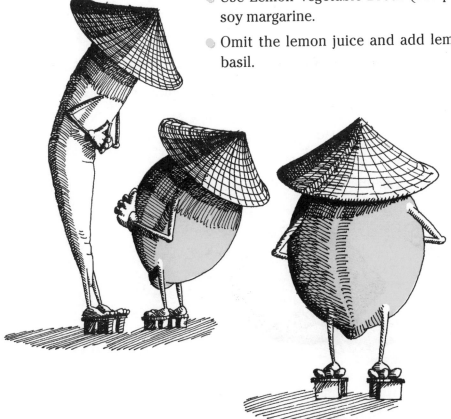

Slivers of Lemon and Broccoli

A colorful contrast of bright green broccoli and brilliant yellow lemon zest.

1 pound broccoli, trimmed and cut into pieces

2 teaspoons Mock Lemon Butter (see page 235)

½ teaspoon dried marjoram

2 thin lemon slices, cut into slivers

¼ teaspoon freshly ground black pepper

SERVES: 4   PREPARATION TIME: 15 MINUTES

1 Steam the broccoli for 2 to 3 minutes. It should be underdone and very crisp.

2 Melt the Mock Lemon Butter in a large skillet. Add the marjoram and cook for 1 minute over medium heat. Add the lemon slivers and broccoli, and sauté for 3 to 5 minutes.

3 Place the broccoli in a large bowl, toss in the pepper, and serve immediately.

Note From A Healthy Lemon:

The broccoli will soak up the lemon butter as it cooks in the skillet. If the skillet becomes too dry but you want to avoid adding additional fat, simply squeeze some more lemon juice into the pan or add 1 tablespoon Lemon Vegetable Broth (see page 86).

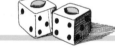

TAKE A CHANCE:

- For an even more colorful presentation, add a diced red bell pepper.
- Add quartered mushrooms or pearl onions.
- Stir in a few drops of hot sauce.
- Sauté with 2 or 3 dried red chili peppers.

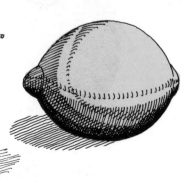

Elegant Lemon Broccoli With Yogurt Cheese Sauce

This dish is great for a special sit-down dinner or on the buffet table because it is just as delicious warm as it is at room temperature. Edible flowers add an elegant touch.

1½ pounds broccoli, trimmed and cut into 3-inch spears

2 tablespoons light sesame or safflower oil

8 ounces small mushrooms, stems removed

1 large red bell pepper, seeded and cut into ½ -inch strips

1 teaspoon dried oregano

1 cup Lemony Yogurt Cheese Spread (see page 236)

2 tablespoons soymilk

6 drops hot chili pepper sauce

juice of 2 medium lemons

10 edible flower heads such as nasturtiums

SERVES: 4   PREPARATION TIME: 20 MINUTES

1 Steam the broccoli for 5 minutes. It should still be crisp and dark green.

2 Heat the oil in a medium-sized skillet. Add the mushrooms and sauté for 3 minutes over medium heat. Add the red pepper strips and oregano, and continue cooking for another 3 minutes. The vegetables should be crisp and colorful.

3 Slightly warm the yogurt cheese spread in the top of a simmering double boiler. Add the soymilk and hot pepper sauce, and simmer for 1 minute. Do not boil.

4 Toss the broccoli with the lemon juice and mound in the center of a large flat serving dish. Alternately place a slice of red pepper and a mushroom cap around the border of the dish. Pour the yogurt sauce over the top of the broccoli, garnish with the nasturtiums, and serve.

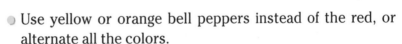

TAKE A CHANCE:

- Use yellow or orange bell peppers instead of the red, or alternate all the colors.

- Use lemon basil instead of the oregano.

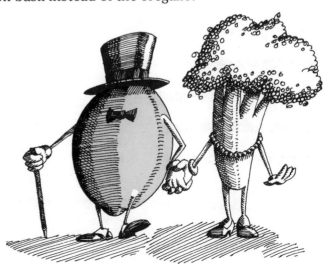

Parsley Potatoes With Mock Lemon Butter

These were always a favorite childhood treat of ours. Too bad we didn't learn about lemon butter until we were grown up.

6 medium white or red potatoes, quartered

3 tablespoons Mock Lemon Butter (see page 235)

3 tablespoons coarsely chopped fresh parsley

SERVES: 4   PREPARATION TIME: 20 MINUTES

1 Place the potatoes in a large pot and cover with water. Bring to a boil. Reduce the heat to medium-high and cook, covered, until the potatoes are soft but not mushy, about 20 minutes. Drain.

2 Transfer the potatoes to a large bowl or platter. Dot the potatoes with the Mock Lemon Butter, garnish with the parsley, and serve immediately.

TAKE A CHANCE:

Use fresh dill or rosemary instead of the parsley.

Add sautéed sliced mushrooms or peas to the potatoes.

Use Herbed Mock Lemon Butter (see page 235).

If you don't have any Mock Lemon Butter on hand, just add the grated zest and juice of 1 medium lemon and 3 tablespoons soy margarine to the cooked potatoes.

Lemonaid

Add a few drops of lemon juice to the cooking water to help vegetables retain their bright colors and to keep white vegetables looking white.

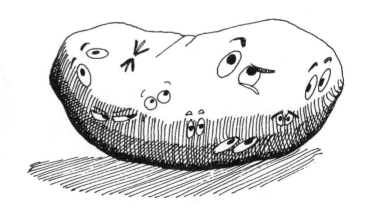

Baked Potatoes With Almost Sour Cream

everything we usually put on baked potatoes is bad for us. Well, just about everything. Almost Sour Cream is so delicious on a baked potato, you won't even know it's not the real thing.

4 baking potatoes, scrubbed

1 cup Almost Sour Cream (see page 234)

$\frac{1}{4}$ teaspoon freshly ground black pepper

$\frac{1}{4}$ cup chopped fresh chives

SERVES: 4   PREPARATION TIME: 1 HOUR

1 Place the potatoes on a cookie sheet and bake in a 350°F oven for about 1 hour, or until soft.

2 Cut the potatoes open down the middle and top with the Almost Sour Cream and a sprinkling of the pepper and chives. Serve immediately.

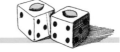

TAKE A CHANCE:

● Add some soy cheese to the potatoes.

● Wrap the potatoes in foil and cook on the grill for about 45 minutes, or until soft.

● Use dill instead of the chives.

● Omit the Almost Sour Cream and use Fresh Lemony Salsa (see page 59) or Colorful Stir-Fry Peppers (see page 174).

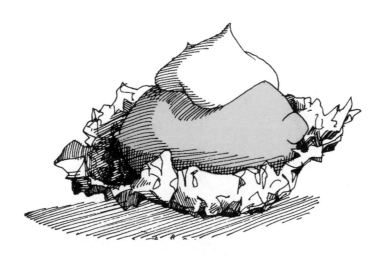

Lemon Lover's Mashed Potatoes

Try this version of mashed potatoes and you'll never return to mere butter-and-milk potatoes again. You won't even need gravy!

4 large potatoes, peeled and cut into pieces

juice of 2 medium lemons

2 tablespoons extra virgin olive oil

$\frac{1}{2}$ teaspoon freshly ground black pepper

Lemonaid

When measuring grated zest in a spoon, pack it loosely.

SERVES: 4   PREPARATION TIME: 30 MINUTES

1 Place the potatoes in a large pot and cover with water. Simmer, covered, until tender, about 20 minutes.

2 Drain the potatoes and mash with the remaining ingredients until smooth. Serve immediately.

Note From a Healthy Lemon:

Cook and mash the potatoes with their skins on. This not only adds a little texture to the potatoes but also retains the vitamins contained in the peel.

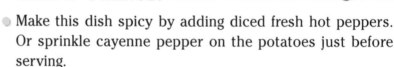

TAKE A CHANCE:

• Make this dish spicy by adding diced fresh hot peppers. Or sprinkle cayenne pepper on the potatoes just before serving.

• Add ½ cup finely minced onion.

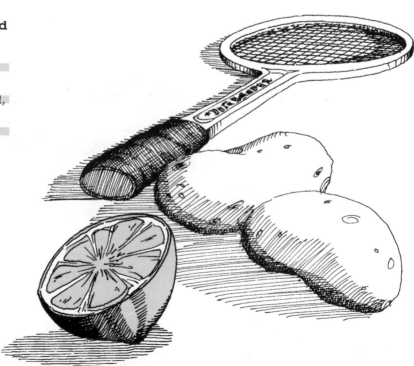

Sweets With Mock Lemon Butter

Many cooks believe that sweet potatoes should be served only at Thanksgiving and Christmas with marshmallows and gobs of brown sugar. Not true! These sweet treats are available all year-round and are just perfect for the lemon lover's taste.

4 medium sweet potatoes, cut into $\frac{1}{2}$-inch slices

2 tablespoons Mock Lemon Butter (see page 235)

grated zest and juice of 1 medium lemon

$\frac{1}{2}$ teaspoon freshly ground black pepper

SERVES: 4 PREPARATION TIME: 40 MINUTES

1 Place the potatoes in a large pot and cover with water. Simmer, covered, until tender, about 15 minutes. Drain and peel.

2 Melt the butter in a large skillet over low heat. Add the lemon zest, lemon juice, and potato slices, and sauté until a light brown crust forms on each side, about 20 minutes. Sprinkle with the pepper and toss.

3 Place the sweets in a large dish with any butter remaining in the skillet and serve immediately.

TAKE A CHANCE:

● Use yams instead of the sweet potatoes.

● Instead of boiling, cook the whole sweet potatoes in a microwave oven for 5 to 7 minutes, or until soft. Then slice and sauté.

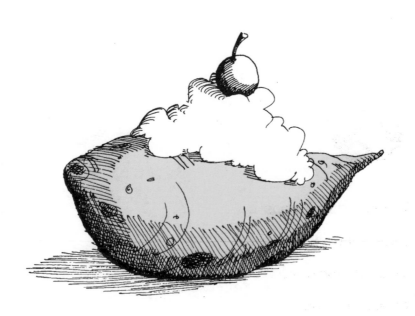

Colorful Stir-Fry Peppers

*Y*ou will be pleased to put these purposefully piquant peppers on your plate.

2 teaspoons light sesame or safflower oil

½ medium purple onion, cut lengthwise into ¼-inch strips

2 teaspoons Lemon Vegetable Broth (see page 86)

juice of 1 medium lemon

2 red bell peppers, seeded and cut into ¼-inch strips

2 yellow bell peppers, seeded and cut into ¼-inch strips

2 green bell peppers, seeded and cut into ¼-inch strips

2 Anaheim chili peppers, seeded and cut into ¼-inch strips

2 teaspoons sesame seeds

SERVES: 4   PREPARATION TIME: 20 MINUTES

1 Heat the oil in a large skillet and sauté the onion for 2 minutes over medium heat. Add all the remaining ingredients except the sesame seeds and sauté for another 5 minutes. The peppers should retain their shape.

2 Place the vegetables in a large dish, garnish with the sesame seeds, and serve immediately.

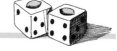

TAKE A CHANCE:

- Add the grated zest of 1 lemon.
- Let the peppers cook until they are soft, then serve them over baked potatoes.
- Add a few jalapeño peppers for some spice.
- Use black sesame seeds.

Lemonaid

When a dish "needs something," the acid in lemon juice will perk it right up.

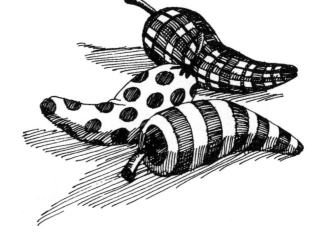

Saucy Lemon Asparagus Bundles

This is a colorful culinary presentation for your family and friends.

1 pound asparagus, trimmed

¾ cup plus 2 tablespoons Lemon Vegetable Broth (see page 86)

½ large red bell pepper, seeded and cut into ¼-inch strips

grated zest and juice of 1 medium lemon

1 teaspoon arrowroot

2 teaspoons finely minced fresh parsley

¼ teaspoon freshly ground black pepper

zest of 1 medium lemon, cut in one continuous strip

SERVES: 4 PREPARATION TIME: 20 MINUTES

1 Steam the asparagus until tender, or cook in a small amount of boiling water in a large pot for about 6 minutes.

2 Heat 2 tablespoons of the broth in a small skillet and sauté the red pepper strips over medium heat until soft.

3 Mix the grated zest and remaining broth in a small bowl. Combine 1 tablespoon of the broth with the arrowroot and mix well. Gradually add the arrowroot to the remaining broth, mix well, and add to the skillet. Bring to a boil and stir constantly until the mixture thickens. Remove from the heat and stir in the lemon juice, parsley, and black pepper.

4 Pour half of the sauce into the bottom of a flat serving dish. Make individual bundles of the asparagus and wrap them with a red pepper strip. Place the bundles on top of the sauce. Then place a piece of the continuous strip of lemon zest over the red pepper and cut to size. Serve the remaining sauce on the side.

TAKE A CHANCE:

• Omit the red bell pepper and tie each bundle with a ribbon of lemon zest. As you remove the asparagus from the steamer or pan, drop the strip of lemon zest into the pan for a second or two. This will make it easier to tie into a bow.

• Omit the sauce and don't make bundles. Just sprinkle the vegetables with lemon. Of course, then you can eat the asparagus the proper way—with your fingers!

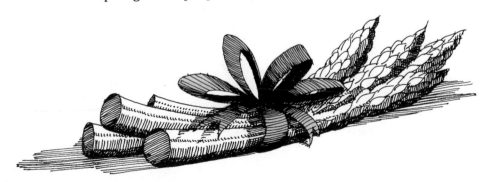

*A*rtichokes à la Caesar

These lemony artichokes are delicious as part of a special luncheon.

juice of 2 medium lemons (reserve the lemon hulls)

2 large garlic cloves, crushed

½ cup minced fresh parsley

4 teaspoons extra virgin olive oil

2 teaspoons grated Parmesan or tofu-Parmesan cheese

¼ teaspoon freshly ground black pepper

4 medium artichokes

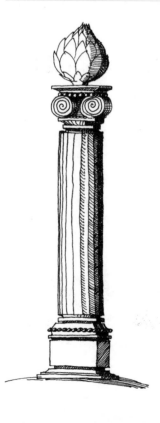

SERVES: 4   PREPARATION TIME: 45 MINUTES

1 Mix all the ingredients except the lemon hulls and artichokes in a small bowl. Cover and let sit at room temperature for 30 minutes.

2 Using a sharp knife, cut the top leaves off the artichokes about 1 inch down. Discard any small leaves at the base and trim the stems flush with the bottoms so the artichokes will stand upright. Using scissors, snip off all the thorn-like leaf ends. Using the juiced lemon hulls, rub the artichokes to prevent discoloration.

3 Place the artichokes upside down in a large pot containing 1½ inches of water, cover, and steam for 30 minutes, or until tender. Check the water to be sure it doesn't evaporate, adding more as necessary. Drain the artichokes upside down in a strainer until cool enough to handle.

4 Spread the artichoke leaves and remove the light green leaves in the center. Using a spoon, scrape out the tough choke at the center of the artichoke and discard.

5 Place each artichoke on an individual serving plate and pour the dressing over the top. These artichokes may be served warm or at room temperature. Have some crusty Italian bread on hand to soak up the wonderful dressing.

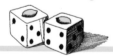

TAKE A CHANCE:

● Add fresh mint, basil, or oregano to the dressing.

● Sprinkle Lemon Garlic Croutons (see page 225) over the artichokes before serving.

● Instead of steaming the artichokes on the stove top, place them in a covered dish or wrap them in waxed paper, and microwave for 4 to 6 minutes, or until tender.

Black Beans With Lemon Slices

Black beans have a wonderful flavor and a velvety texture. Try these beans as is with Citrus Vegetable Fajitas (see page 115), or purée them and spread on a warm tortilla.

1 pound dried black beans, sorted and rinsed

4 cups water

1 tablespoon safflower oil

$\frac{1}{2}$ medium lemon, thinly sliced

1 large onion, coarsely chopped

4 large garlic cloves, minced

2 large red or green jalapeño peppers, coarsely chopped

2 tablespoons chopped fresh cilantro

Lemonaid

Keep vegetables and fruits from discoloring by rubbing with a lemon slice or dipping in a bath of four parts water and one part lemon juice.

S E R V E S : 4 P R E P A R A T I O N T I M E : 2 4 H O U R S

1 Place the beans in a large pot with enough water to completely cover them. Soak overnight at room temperature. Don't drain off the water.

2 Add the 4 cups water to the bean pot, place over medium heat, and simmer, covered, for 1½ hours, or until the beans are tender.

3 Heat the oil in a small skillet and sauté the lemon slices, onion, garlic, and jalapeños over medium heat for 3 minutes. Add the sauté mixture to the beans and continue to simmer for 30 minutes. If the beans contain extra liquid when they are finished cooking, turn the heat to high and cook, stirring constantly, until the liquid is reduced.

4 Place the beans in a large bowl, garnish with the cilantro, and serve immediately.

TAKE A CHANCE:

● Make refried black beans by heating the cooked beans in a large skillet over medium-high heat. Lightly mash the beans with a fork, adding 2 teaspoons olive oil.

● Use pinto beans instead of the black beans, or mix them half and half.

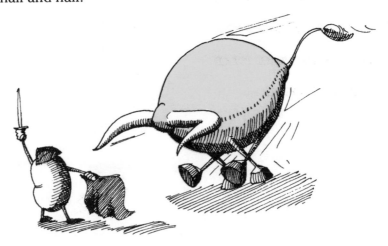

Green Beans With Lemon and Garlic

These beans are cooked twice, both steamed and sautéed, but should still be crisp when served.

1 pound green beans, trimmed and cut into 2-inch lengths

2 teaspoons extra virgin olive oil

2 large garlic cloves, finely minced

juice of 1 medium lemon

8 fresh lemon thyme leaves, chopped

Lemonaid

Add a bit of lemon thyme or a handful of thick lemon slices to your bath water for a soothing scent.

SERVES: 4   PREPARATION TIME: 15 MINUTES

1 Steam the beans for 2 minutes. They should still be crisp when they are snapped.

2 Heat the oil in a large skillet and sauté the garlic for 1 minute over medium heat. Add the beans and cook for 1 minute more, stirring constantly. Add the lemon juice and cook for 2 more minutes.

3 Place the beans in a large bowl, sprinkle them with the lemon thyme, and serve immediately.

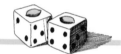

TAKE A CHANCE:

● Stir in 8 ounces sliced mushrooms.

● Sprinkle the beans with toasted almond slices before serving.

● Use crisp steamed broccoli instead of the green beans.

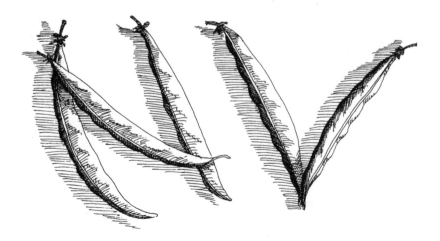

Grilled Herbed Corn on the Cob

Nothing beats fresh corn from the garden, especially when it's dressed with lemon.

4 ears fresh corn, husked and trimmed

2 teaspoons Mock Lemon Butter (see page 235), at room temperature

¼ teaspoon freshly ground black pepper

SERVES: 4   PREPARATION TIME: 30 MINUTES

1 Cut 4 squares of aluminum foil, 12-x-12-inches each, and place one ear of corn in the center of each square.

2 Spread an equal amount of Mock Lemon Butter on each ear of corn and sprinkle with the pepper.

3 Fold the aluminum foil into a packet around each ear of corn, making sure to crimp the edges tightly. Place the packets on a hot grill and close the lid. Turn the corn several times during cooking. Depending on the type of grill used and the freshness of the corn, the corn should take about 15 minutes to cook.

4 Place the packets on individual plates and serve with any remaining butter. Remember to warn everyone to be careful of squirting hot butter when cutting into the packets.

Note From a Healthy Lemon:

The rich lemony taste of the Mock Lemon Butter should eliminate or cut down on the salt normally used on roasted corn. If you want to eliminate the fat, too, try sprinkling the corn with just lemon juice or grated lemon zest with pepper before grilling.

TAKE A CHANCE:

- Omit the lemon juice and place lemon mint, lemon balm, or lemon verbena on the Mock Lemon Butter.
- Omit the Mock Lemon Butter and wrap slices of lemon in with the corn. Serve with soy margarine on the side.

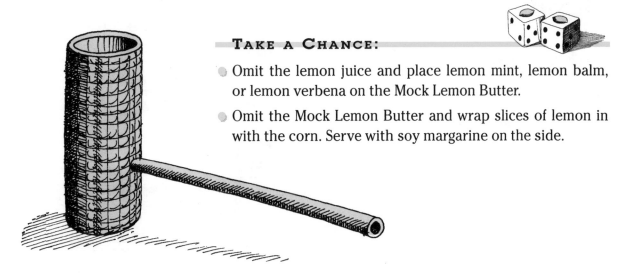

Lemony Garlic Mushrooms

This wonderful mushroom dish can be prepared in a flash and can be served as a side dish or an appetizer. Make it ahead of time and serve it barely warm as an elegant addition to any meal.

1 pound mushrooms

2 tablespoons extra virgin olive oil

3 large garlic cloves, thinly sliced

juice of 2 medium lemons

$\frac{1}{2}$ cup water

$\frac{1}{2}$ teaspoon crushed red pepper

freshly ground black pepper to taste

Lemonaid

Use lemon tree leaves as doilies beneath the small appetizer dishes that sit on top of your larger serving trays.

SERVES: 4   PREPARATION TIME: 20 MINUTES

1 Quarter the mushrooms if they are large. If they are small, leave them whole.

2 Heat the oil in a small skillet and sauté the garlic for 1 minute over medium heat. Do not brown the garlic. Add the mushrooms and sauté for 2 minutes. If the garlic starts to brown, remove it and add fresh garlic.

3 Add the lemon juice, water, and red pepper to the mushrooms. Lower the heat and simmer for 2 minutes. Add the black pepper to taste.

4 Transfer the mushrooms to a large bowl and serve them hot or only warm. Accompany this dish with fresh, crusty bread to soak up the juices.

TAKE A CHANCE:

- Stir in 2 tablespoons minced fresh parsley before serving.
- Use whole dried red chili peppers instead of the crushed red pepper.
- Add more red pepper.

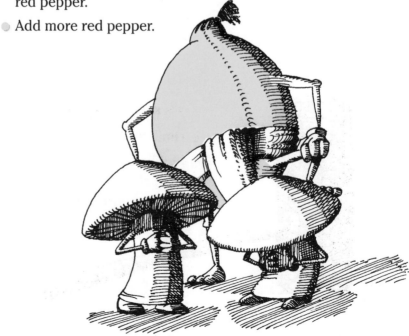

Luscious Brussels Sprouts

P op one of these little green morsels in your mouth and bite down on a tasty surprise.

2 cups Brussels sprouts, trimmed

$\frac{1}{4}$ cup Lemon Vegetable Broth (see page 86)

grated zest and juice of 1 medium lemon

$\frac{1}{4}$ teaspoon freshly ground black pepper

1 teaspoon soy margarine

$\frac{1}{2}$ cup whole wheat bread crumbs

S E R V E S : 4   P R E P A R A T I O N   T I M E : 20 M I N U T E S

1 Cut a small X into the stem of each Brussels sprout with a sharp knife. This will accelerate the cooking time.

2 Heat the broth, lemon zest, lemon juice, and pepper in a small saucepan. Add the Brussels sprouts, stir, cover, and simmer over low heat until the sprouts are tender, about 10 minutes.

3 In a small skillet, melt the margarine. Add the bread crumbs and stir until the margarine is absorbed.

4 Place the sprouts in a small serving bowl with the pan liquid and sprinkle with the bread crumbs. Serve immediately.

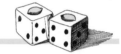

TAKE A CHANCE:

● Add 1 small sliced carrot.

● Sprinkle with caraway seeds.

Lemonaid

Wrap lemon halves in cheesecloth to direct the lemon juice where you want it to go when squeezed and to keep the seeds out of the dish.

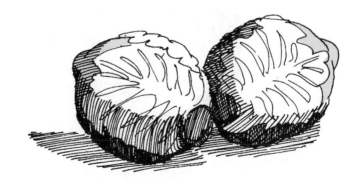

Braised Lemon Cabbage

Although we use cabbage as a staple to help get us through the long winter, this version is best when the cabbage is fresh from the garden in spring.

¼ cup Lemon Vegetable Broth (see page 86)

¼ cup diced onion

½ large head cabbage, cut into ¼-inch slices

grated zest and juice of 1 medium lemon

⅛ teaspoon freshly ground black pepper

SERVES: 4   PREPARATION TIME: 20 MINUTES

1 Heat the broth in a medium skillet. Add the onion and sauté for 1 minute. Add the cabbage, cover, and cook until wilted, about 5 minutes.

2 Place the cabbage in a large serving bowl, add the lemon zest, lemon juice, and black pepper, and toss. Serve immediately.

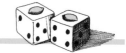

TAKE A CHANCE:

● Sauté ½ cup whole wheat bread crumbs in 2 teaspoons soy margarine and sprinkle on top of the cabbage.

● Use Chinese cabbage.

● Add ½ cup sliced red cabbage.

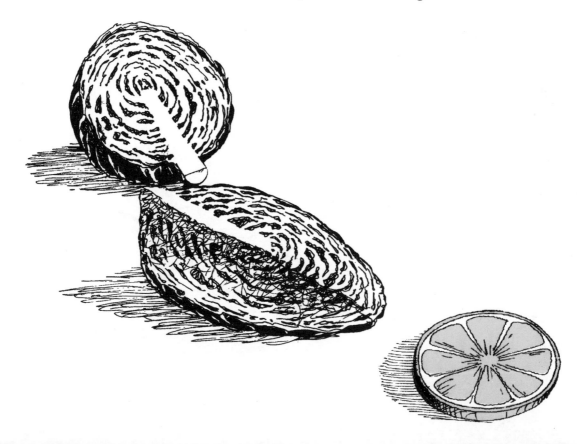

Lemon Mint Zucchini

This tart and tangy dish can be prepared in advance and used as a side dish or appetizer.

2 teaspoons extra virgin olive oil

6 small zucchini, cut into $\frac{1}{8}$-inch slices

3 tablespoons lemon juice

2 tablespoons coarsely chopped fresh lemon mint

$\frac{1}{4}$ teaspoon Lemon Pepper (see page 227)

SERVES: 6   PREPARATION TIME: 15 MINUTES

1 Heat the oil in a large skillet and sauté the zucchini until golden on both sides. Remove the zucchini with a slotted spoon and drain on paper toweling.

2 Place the zucchini on a large platter and pour the lemon juice over it. Sprinkle with the lemon mint and Lemon Pepper.

3 Cool the zucchini to room temperature and serve.

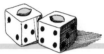

TAKE A CHANCE:

- Drizzle with extra olive oil before adding the lemon and mint.

- Sauté with slices of red bell pepper for extra color.

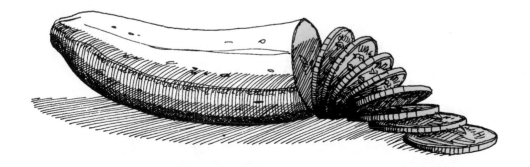

Zucchini Lemon Sauté

A tasty way to use the bounty of your summer garden. Buy a tube of tomato paste for recipes that call for small amounts.

2 teaspoons safflower oil

1 large garlic clove, finely minced

4 small zucchini, cut into ½-inch slices

2 tablespoons tomato paste

juice of 1 medium lemon

2 teaspoons chopped fresh oregano, or 1 teaspoon dried

Lemonaid

Lemon juice will work as a bleach in your washing machine. It'll make your clothes smell great, too. Add a cup to the water after the wash cycle begins.

SERVES: 4 PREPARATION TIME: 20 MINUTES

1 Heat the oil in a large skillet and sauté the garlic for 1 minute over medium heat. Add the zucchini and sauté for 2 to 3 minutes, stirring constantly.

2 Add the tomato paste to the zucchini and cook for 5 minutes. The zucchini should still be slightly crisp. Add the lemon juice and oregano, and stir for another minute.

3 Place the zucchini in a large bowl and serve immediately.

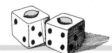

TAKE A CHANCE:

- Mix in a small amount of diced eggplant.
- Use crookneck squash with or instead of the zucchini.
- Add a few sliced mushrooms.

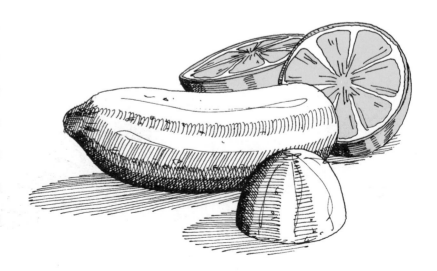

Zippy Roasted Vegetables

*R*oasting vegetables instead of stewing or sautéing gives them an entirely different flavor. The aroma brings back the smell of Sunday dinner slowly cooking in the oven.

---

juice of 1½ medium lemons

5 large garlic cloves, crushed

½ cup Lemon Vegetable Broth (see page 86)

2 tablespoons canola oil

8 small red potatoes, quartered

2 large zucchini, quartered

3 large carrots, quartered

1 large onion, cut lengthwise into eighths

1½ teaspoons finely chopped fresh rosemary, or 2 teaspoons dried

2 teaspoons finely minced fresh parsley

SERVES: 4   PREPARATION TIME: 45 MINUTES

1 Place ¼ cup of the lemon juice and all of the garlic, broth, and oil in a small saucepan and simmer for 1 minute over medium heat.

2 Place the vegetables in a 2-quart baking dish, pour the broth over the top, and toss until the vegetables are well coated. Cover the pan tightly with a lid or aluminum foil and bake in a 350°F oven for 20 minutes.

3 Remove the cover from the vegetables and add the rosemary, mixing well. Return the uncovered vegetables to the oven until all the vegetables are cooked, approximately 20 to 25 minutes.

4 Place the vegetables in a large dish. Add the remaining lemon juice to the broth in the baking dish and stir. Pour the broth over the vegetables, garnish with the parsley, and serve immediately.

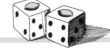

TAKE A CHANCE:

● Toss the finished vegetables with 1 tablespoon grated lemon zest.

● Use oregano or dill instead of the rosemary.

● Bake 3 or 4 lemon slices with the vegetables.

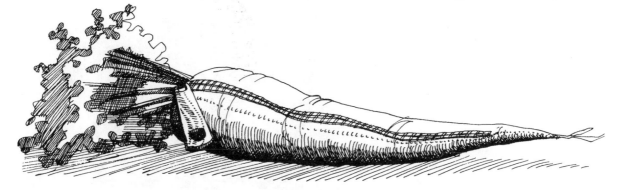

Steamed Vegetable Medley With Lemon and Shoyu

Lemon and shoyu sauce give these vegetables an *exotic oriental flavor.*

1 large potato, peeled and cut into ½-inch slices

1 large sweet potato, peeled and cut into ½-inch slices

2 large broccoli stalks, chopped into 2-inch pieces

8 ounces green beans, trimmed and cut into 2-inch pieces

2 medium zucchini, cut into ½-inch slices

1 large carrot, peeled and cut into ½-inch slices

1 medium turnip, peeled and cut into ½-inch slices

1 small eggplant, peeled and cut into ½-inch cubes

grated zest and juice of 1 medium lemon

½ teaspoon date sugar

3 tablespoons shoyu or tamari sauce

SERVES: 4   PREPARATION TIME: 30 MINUTES

1 Layer the potatoes in a steamer and cook for 5 minutes.

2 Add the remaining vegetables to the steamer and cook until done, about 10 minutes. They should be tender but not mushy.

3 Mix the lemon zest, lemon juice, date sugar, and shoyu or tamari sauce in a small bowl until the sugar dissolves. Toss the vegetables with the dressing and serve immediately.

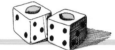

TAKE A CHANCE:

● Use honey instead of the date sugar.

● Add 1 teaspoon hot chili paste to the dressing.

● Cut all the vegetables into a medium dice and steam for only 2 to 3 minutes. Serve over a bed of lettuce with the dressing on the side.

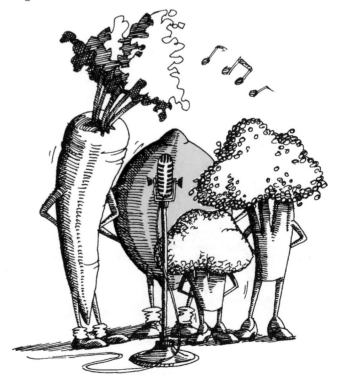

Lemon-Showered Vegetable Ragout

A squirt of lemon juice on top of simmered vegetables adds a wonderfully refreshing tang. This recipe is limited only by the vegetables available in the grocery store. Mix and match your favorites, but don't forget the lemon! Serve with crusty bread or tuck inside a warm pita.

¼ cup Lemon Vegetable Broth (see page 86)

1 medium onion, finely chopped

2 large garlic cloves, finely minced

8 ounces large mushrooms, trimmed and quartered

2 small zucchini, cut into ½-inch slices

2 small crookneck squash, cut into ½-inch slices

1 small green bell pepper, seeded and cut into ¼-inch slices

1 small eggplant, peeled and cut into ½-inch cubes

3 large tomatoes, chopped

1 teaspoon freshly ground black pepper

juice of 1 medium lemon

SERVES: 4   PREPARATION TIME: 45 MINUTES

1 Heat the broth in a large skillet. Add the onion and sauté for 2 minutes over high heat. Add the garlic and sauté for another minute. Add all the remaining ingredients except the lemon juice, cover, and reduce the heat to medium. Simmer for 25 minutes, stirring occasionally. Check the level of liquid in the pan frequently, adding more broth if the vegetables seem dry.

2 Transfer the vegetables to a large bowl. Add the lemon juice, mix, and serve immediately.

TAKE A CHANCE:

● If you would like more sauce for your vegetables, add ½ cup to 1 cup tomato sauce to the vegetables.

● Serve over rice, pasta, or couscous.

● Spice things up by adding 1 or 2 chopped jalapeño peppers.

● Sprinkle with freshly grated Parmesan or tofu-Parmesan cheese.

● Add 1 teaspoon oregano or marjoram.

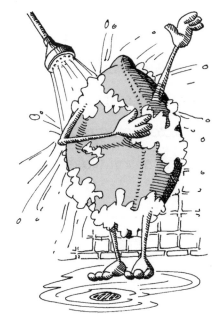

7angy Minted Peas

*N*o one will say they don't like peas after tasting *these tangy, herbed beauties.*

2 cups green peas

10 large fresh mint leaves, finely chopped

juice of 1 medium lemon

SERVES: 4   PREPARATION TIME: 10 MINUTES

1 Place the peas in a small saucepan in a small amount of water. Cover and cook over medium heat for 3 to 4 minutes, or until tender. Drain.

2 Transfer the peas to a small bowl, toss with the mint and lemon juice, and serve immediately.

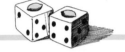

TAKE A CHANCE:

- Use frozen peas instead of the fresh.
- Omit the lemon juice and add lemon mint, lemon sage, or lemon basil.
- Use regular basil, dill, oregano, or sage.
- Add 1 teaspoon Herbed Mock Lemon Butter (see page 235).
- Add grated lemon zest.

Lemonaid

Gargle with lemon juice if you have a sore throat. It's easier to take than a glass of warm salt water.

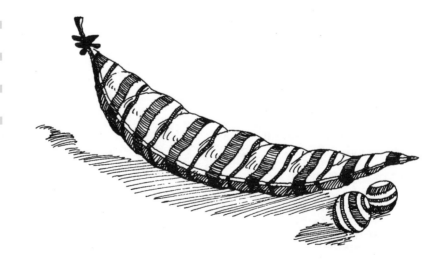

Chapter 9

Desserts and Snacks— A Lemony Treat

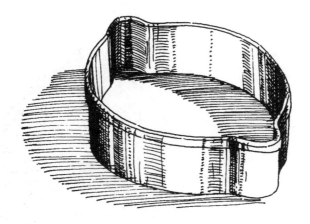

emons make tempting desserts and snacks even more tempting with a tart taste that keeps everyone satisfied. Our recipes include some very healthy treats that are also wickedly delicious. If any of the recipes has more sweetness or eggs than you like in your diet, try one of the many guiltless goodies we've concocted for you.

Salted Lemons

Under the scorching sun of the vast Southwest desert, children of all ages quench their thirst by sucking on these lemons. The whole lemon is eaten, skin and all. Beware—this recipe is high in salt, so make it only on occasion.

4 salted plums (available in the Latin American section of most grocery stores)

2 medium lemons, cut in half

SERVES: 4   PREPARATION TIME: 1 MINUTE

1 Place a salted plum in the center of each lemon half.

2 Wrap a napkin around each lemon half and serve.

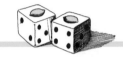

TAKE A CHANCE:

◦ Place a salted plum on one half of the lemon and cover it with the other half. Wrap the lemon in plastic wrap and let sit at room temperature for 1 hour. Remove the wrap and serve. This will reduce the salty taste and allow the salt to permeate the whole lemon.

Lemonaid

The largest harvests of fresh lemons occur in the late summer and mid-winter. Plan your recipes accordingly.

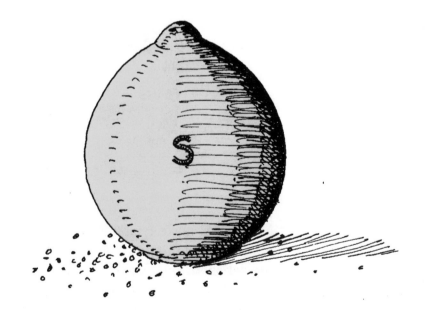

Creamy Lemon Papaya

A simple, elegant, refreshing dessert that makes a very exotic presentation.

grated zest and juice of 1 medium lemon

1 teaspoon malt powder

2 large egg yolks

8 ounces silken tofu

2 medium papayas, cut in half and seeded

4 fresh mint sprigs

SERVES: 4   PREPARATION TIME: 45 MINUTES

1 Place the lemon zest, lemon juice, malt powder, and egg yolks in a large bowl and mix until the sugar dissolves. Set aside.

2 Using a spoon, mash the tofu in a small bowl. Gently fold the tofu into the lemon juice mixture. Cover and refrigerate for 30 minutes.

3 Mound the lemon cream in the center of each papaya half, garnish with the mint, and serve.

TAKE A CHANCE:

- Use lemon mint instead of the regular mint.
- Instead of mixing the grated lemon zest into the cream, sprinkle it on top as a garnish.
- Omit the lemon cream and just sprinkle lemon juice on the papaya.
- Decorate the serving plate with leaves from your lemon tree.

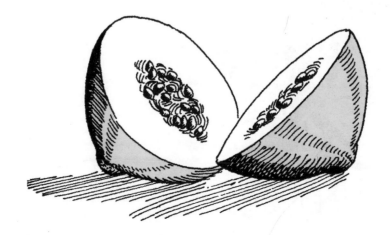

Simple Lemon Custard

A thick and creamy custard with a fresh lemon taste.

grated zest and juice of 1 medium lemon

3 large eggs

2 cups soymilk

2 tablespoons date sugar

SERVES: 4   PREPARATION TIME: 1 HOUR

1 In a large bowl, whisk together all the ingredients until smooth.

2 Pour the mixture into individual custard cups and place the cups in a pan filled with hot water to within ½ inch of the tops of the cups. Bake in a 350°F oven for 40 to 45 minutes, or until a knife inserted in the center comes out clean. Serve warm or cold.

Note From a Healthy Lemon:

Use a vegetable-based egg substitute instead of the eggs.

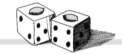

TAKE A CHANCE:

- Sprinkle the custard with a dash of cinnamon or nutmeg before serving.
- Place fruit, like berries or sliced peaches, in the bottom of the custard cups before filling. Serve warm.
- Add 1 teaspoon lemon thyme to the recipe.

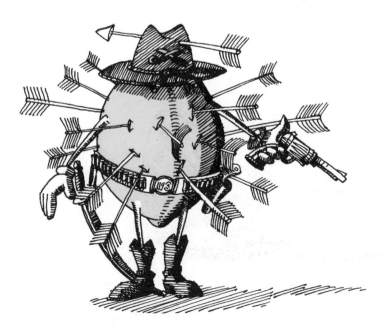

Lemon Strawberry Sherbet

A few tablespoons of sherbet between courses cleanses the palate of lingering aftertastes and gets the mouth ready for the next delicious course.

juice of 3 medium lemons

1 cup puréed strawberries

4 cups soymilk

4 fresh mint sprigs

SERVES: 4 PREPARATION TIME: 6½ HOURS

1 Mix all the ingredients except the mint in an 8-inch-square baking pan. The soymilk may look curdled, but this will disappear in freezing. Cover and freeze until partially frozen, approximately 2 hours.

2 Scrape down the sides of the pan and stir the partially frozen mixture with a spoon. Cover and return to the freezer until firm.

3 Scoop the sherbet into serving dishes, garnish with the mint, and serve immediately.

TAKE A CHANCE:

- To give the sherbet a smoother texture, when removing it from the freezer after the first 2 hours, place the frozen mixture in a medium-sized mixing bowl and beat with a mixer until smooth. Then return to the pan, cover, and freeze until firm.
- Serve in Lemon Cups (see page 195).
- Use raspberries instead of the strawberries.

Lemonaid

When using dried lemon zest instead of fresh zest, adjust the amount to the recipe. More will be needed to approach the flavor intensity of fresh.

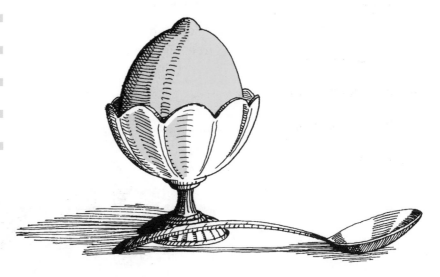

Homemade Lemon Ice Milk

At one time, the old standby was vanilla ice cream. No more! This lemon treat takes only a few hours to make and doesn't even need an ice cream machine.

4 cups soymilk

1 teaspoon vanilla extract

1 tablespoon agar-agar flakes

$\frac{3}{4}$ cup date sugar

3 tablespoons arrowroot

$\frac{2}{3}$ cup lemon juice

$\frac{1}{4}$ cup grated lemon zest

12 fresh mint leaves

Lemonaid

One medium lemon yields about 3 or 4 teaspoons of grated lemon zest.

SERVES: 4   PREPARATION TIME: 5 HOURS

1 Place 2 cups of the soymilk and all of the vanilla, agar-agar, and date sugar in a large saucepan and bring to a boil over high heat. Reduce the heat to low and simmer until the agar-agar flakes have dissolved, about 5 minutes.

2 Dissolve the arrowroot in the remaining 2 cups of soymilk. Add the arrowroot mixture to the agar mixture in the pan and simmer for 2 to 3 minutes, or until the combined mixture starts to thicken.

3 Remove the mixture from the heat, add the lemon juice and lemon zest, and stir well.

4 Pour the lemon mixture into an 8-inch-square pan. Cover and freeze until solid.

5 When the ice milk is solidly frozen, break it up and place pieces in a food processor. Whip the mixture, scraping the sides of the processing container often. Transfer to individual dessert bowls, garnish with the mint, and serve immediately.

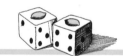

TAKE A CHANCE:

● Add 1 tablespoon chopped lemon or cherry pieces before freezing.

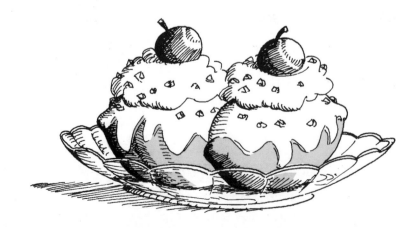

Lemon Ice

C ool, tart, refreshing, and so very, very lemony.

¼ cup malt powder

¼ cup mild honey

4 cups boiling water

grated zest and juice of 6 medium lemons

4 fresh mint sprigs

SERVES: 4   PREPARATION TIME: 6 HOURS

1 Mix the malt powder and honey in a large bowl, add the boiling water, and stir until the honey is dissolved. Cool.

2 Add the lemon zest and lemon juice to the honey mixture and mix well. Pour into an 8-inch-square baking pan, cover, and freeze until partially frozen, approximately 2 hours.

3 Scrape down the sides of the pan and stir the partially frozen mixture with a spoon. Re-cover the pan and return it to the freezer until firm.

4 Scoop the ice into dessert dishes or Lemon Cups (see Take a Chance, below), garnish with the mint, and serve immediately.

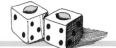

TAKE A CHANCE

Lemon Cups are fun to make and use, and are very aromatic. First, cut 2 lemons in half and squeeze out the juice. Then, use a paring knife to remove the remaining crushed pulp and membrane from the lemon hulls and cut the dimpled ends from the hulls so the Lemon Cups will sit upright. Finally, fill each Lemon Cup with Lemon Ice, ice milk, or your favorite pudding, and serve.

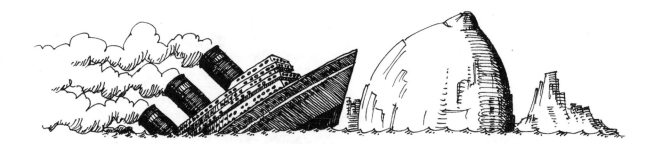

Lemon Snowballs With Minted Raspberry Sauce

Whether summer or winter, you won't mind getting hit with this snowball. This version of mousse uses egg whites instead of high-fat whipping cream.

Snowballs

3 teaspoons unflavored gelatin

¼ cup cold water

grated zest and juice of 1 medium lemon

3 tablespoons malt powder

1 cup boiling water

2 large egg whites, at room temperature

Sauce

1 pint fresh raspberries, hulled

2 tablespoons lemon juice

1 tablespoon concentrated fruit sweetener

¼ cup fresh mint leaves

SERVES: 6   PREPARATION TIME: 3 HOURS

1 To make the snowballs, place the gelatin in the cold water in a large mixing bowl, stir, and let sit for 10 minutes. Add the lemon zest, lemon juice, malt powder, and boiling water. Cover and chill just until the mixture is set, about 1 hour.

2 With an electric mixer, beat the egg whites until stiff, then gently fold the egg whites into the mousse. Spoon the mixture into dessert bowls and chill until set, about 1 hour.

3 To make the sauce, place all the sauce ingredients in a blender or food processor and pulse until the berries are puréed. Transfer the mixture to a bowl, cover, and chill for 30 minutes.

4 Pour the sauce over the snowballs and serve immediately.

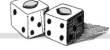

TAKE A CHANCE:

○ Run a hot towel under the dessert bowls and unmold the snowballs onto a serving plate before adding the sauce.

○ Instead of making individual servings, pour the mousse into a 1½-quart mold and chill until firm.

○ Use strawberries or blueberries instead of the raspberries.

○ Top with Fluffy Lemon Topping (see page 242) instead of the Minted Raspberry Sauce.

○ Add 1 teaspoon Sweetened Zest (see page 229) to the egg whites before beating.

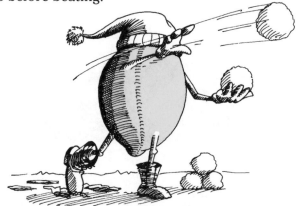

Sinless Lemon Cookies

These cookies are sinfully delicious and only a little bit naughty!

grated zest and juice of 1 medium lemon

1 medium egg

$\frac{1}{4}$ cup concentrated fruit sweetener

$\frac{1}{4}$ cup light sesame or safflower oil

$1\frac{1}{4}$ cups unbleached white or whole wheat pastry flour

$\frac{1}{2}$ teaspoon baking soda

YIELD: 24 COOKIES   PREPARATION TIME: 1 HOUR

1 Place the lemon zest, lemon juice, egg, concentrated fruit sweetener, and oil in a large bowl. Mix well. Add the flour and baking soda, and mix thoroughly.

2 Drop heaping teaspoonfuls of the cookie dough on an ungreased cookie sheet, spacing the cookies 2 inches apart. Bake in a 350°F oven for 5 to 7 minutes, or until light golden brown.

3 Cool completely and serve.

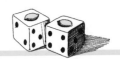

TAKE A CHANCE:

- Omit the lemon zest and add 2 teaspoons dried lemon thyme.

Lemonaid

Lemon thyme can act as a mild deodorant, as an antiseptic, or as a local anesthetic.

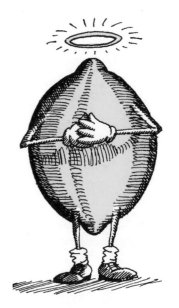

Tangy Gems

light cookies with the fresh sunny taste of lemon.

2 teaspoons lemon juice

grated zest of 2 medium lemons

1 large egg

¼ cup concentrated fruit sweetener

¼ cup safflower oil

1½ cups whole wheat pastry flour

1 teaspoon baking powder

YIELD: 36 COOKIES   PREPARATION TIME: 1 HOUR

1 Place the lemon juice, lemon zest, egg, concentrated fruit sweetener, and oil in a large mixing bowl. Beat the mixture vigorously with a fork. Add the flour and baking powder, and mix thoroughly.

2 Drop teaspoonfuls of the cookie dough on a greased cookie sheet, spacing the cookies 1 inch apart. Flatten each cookie slightly. Bake in a 375°F oven for 8 to 10 minutes, or until lightly browned.

3 Cool completely and serve.

TAKE A CHANCE:

● Sprinkle with Sweetened Zest (see page 229).

● Brush lightly with melted soy margarine while cooling.

● Top with a dot of berry jam after the cookies have cooled.

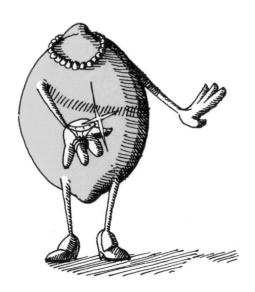

Lemon Snaps

This recipe combines the tart goodness of lemons with another of our favorite childhood cookies. If only someone had thought of this when we were little!

½ cup molasses

1 large egg

½ cup light sesame or safflower oil

grated zest and juice of 1 medium lemon

2½ cups unbleached white flour

½ teaspoon ground ginger

½ teaspoon ground cinnamon

½ teaspoon ground cloves

YIELD: 36 COOKIES   PREPARATION TIME: 2 HOURS

1 Using a spoon, cream the molasses, egg, and oil in a large bowl. Stir in all the remaining ingredients and blend well. Cover and refrigerate for 1 hour.

2 Drop teaspoonfuls of the cookie dough on a lightly greased cookie sheet, spacing the cookies 3 inches apart. Bake in a 375°F oven for 10 to 12 minutes, or until lightly browned.

3 Cool completely and serve.

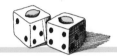

TAKE A CHANCE:

● Use only ¼ teaspoon of each of the ground spices and add additional lemon zest for a more lemony snap.

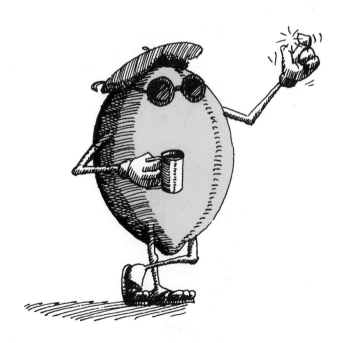

    Lemonaid

Rest your elbows in juiced lemon hulls to remove that hard, dry skin.

Refrigerator Lemon Wafers

Crispy brown edges with a wild tart lemon flavor.

grated zest and juice of 1 medium lemon

$\frac{1}{3}$ cup safflower oil

$\frac{1}{4}$ cup date sugar

1 large egg

1½ cups unbleached white flour

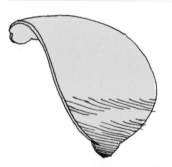

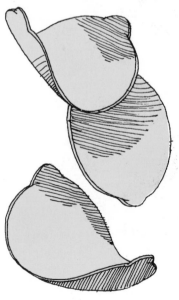

YIELD: 30 COOKIES PREPARATION TIME: 5 HOURS

1 Place all the ingredients except the flour in a large bowl and mix. Gradually add the flour, mixing well.

2 Transfer the dough to a sheet of waxed paper and form into a log 1½ inches in diameter. Wrap the log in the waxed paper and refrigerate for 4 hours.

3 With a sharp knife, cut the log into ¼-inch slices and place the slices 1 inch apart on an ungreased cookie sheet. Bake in a 375°F oven for 10 to 12 minutes, or until lightly browned.

4 Cool completely and serve.

Note From a Healthy Lemon:

Make eggless wafers by using an egg substitute instead of the egg.

TAKE A CHANCE:

● Mix ¼ cup chopped walnuts or almonds into the dough.

Lemondoodles

The rich cinnamon smell of these cookies brings back memories of our childhood. We have enhanced their wonderful taste with the goodness of lemons.

grated zest of 1 medium lemon

1½ teaspoons ground cinnamon

1 tablespoon date sugar

2 tablespoons soy margarine

¼ cup light sesame or safflower oil

3 tablespoons rice syrup

1 large egg

1½ cups whole wheat pastry flour

YIELD: 30 COOKIES   PREPARATION TIME: 30 MINUTES

1 Place the lemon zest, cinnamon, and date sugar in a small bowl and mix. Set aside.

2 Combine all the remaining ingredients in a large bowl, mixing well.

3 Shape rounded teaspoonfuls of the cookie dough into balls and roll in the lemon-cinnamon mixture. Place on an ungreased cookie sheet, spacing the cookies 2 inches apart. Bake in a 375°F oven for 8 minutes, or until the cookies are set.

4 Cool completely and serve.

TAKE A CHANCE:

● Don't waste any leftover lemon-cinnamon mixture. Sprinkle it on sliced apples, or add it to hot tea or Lemon-Kissed Oatmeal (see page 269).

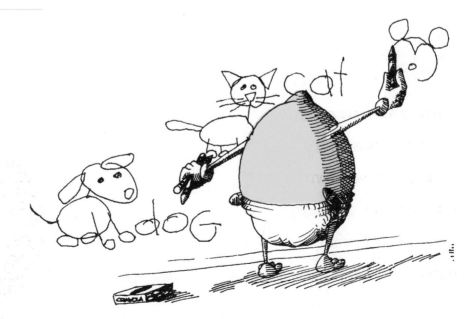

Lemon Cheweys

These crispy delights leave a clean, fresh lemon taste in your mouth. You won't be satisfied until the plate is clean.

---

grated zest and juice of 1 medium lemon

---

2 tablespoons soymilk

¼ cup canola oil

¼ cup malt powder

½ teaspoon vanilla extract

¾ cup unbleached white flour

¾ teaspoon baking powder

YIELD: 24 COOKIES   PREPARATION TIME: 2½ HOURS

1 Place the lemon zest, lemon juice, soymilk, oil, malt powder, and vanilla in a blender or food processor, and process until smooth. Add the flour and baking powder, and pulse 3 to 4 times, or until the mixture is well blended.

2 Transfer the dough to a sheet of waxed paper and form into a log 1½ inches in diameter. Wrap the log in the waxed paper and refrigerate for 2 hours.

3 With a sharp knife, cut the log into ⅛-inch slices and place the slices 2 inches apart on an ungreased cookie sheet. Bake in a 350°F oven for 6 to 8 minutes, or until golden.

4 Cool completely and serve.

TAKE A CHANCE:

● Sprinkle date sugar on top of the cookies when they are removed from the oven.

Lemonaid

Make a formal centerpiece by arranging fruit and leaves from a lemon tree in a fancy low-cut glass bowl.

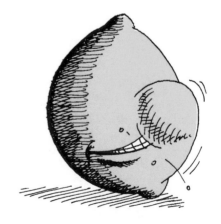

Zesty Gingerbread

There is nothing in the world that brings back childhood memories like the spicy smell of fresh gingerbread. The only thing better is our updated version with lemon-coated raisins.

grated zest of 1 medium lemon

¾ cup dark raisins

2 cups whole wheat pastry flour

1 teaspoon ground cinnamon

1 teaspoon ground ginger

1 teaspoon ground allspice

½ cup soymilk

½ cup molasses

2 tablespoons light sesame or safflower oil

1 large egg

SERVES: 6   PREPARATION TIME: 1 HOUR

1 Toss the lemon zest and raisins together in a small bowl and set aside.

2 Mix the flour and spices together in a large bowl. Set aside.

3 Mix all the remaining ingredients together in a small bowl. Add the liquid mixture to the flour mixture, stirring until just blended.

4 Stir the raisin mixture into the batter. Mix only until the raisins are distributed throughout the batter.

5 Pour the batter into a greased 9-inch-square baking pan and bake in a 350°F oven for 20 minutes, or until a toothpick inserted in the center comes out clean. Cool for at least 20 minutes. Cut into squares and serve.

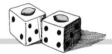

TAKE A CHANCE:

● Use unbleached white flour instead of the whole wheat pastry flour.

● Add ¼ cup chopped walnuts or pecans.

● Serve with Fluffy Lemon Topping (see page 242).

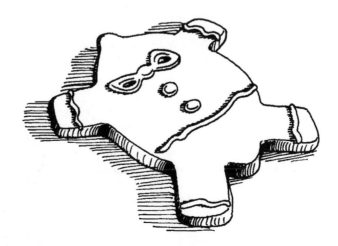

Lemon Sauced Crêpes

These elegant crêpes make an impressive dessert for family or friends.

Sauce

grated zest and juice of 1 medium lemon

2 teaspoons Sucanat

$1\frac{1}{2}$ tablespoons arrowroot

$\frac{1}{4}$ cup water

2 teaspoons melted soy margarine

Crêpes

grated zest of 1 medium lemon

1 cup soymilk

2 large eggs

$\frac{1}{2}$ cup unbleached white flour

1 tablespoon soy margarine

SERVES: 4   PREPARATION TIME: 45 MINUTES

1 To make the sauce, blend all the sauce ingredients except the melted margarine in a small saucepan. Cook over medium-high heat, stirring constantly, until the mixture is thick and has reached a boil.

2 Remove the mixture from the heat and continue stirring for 1 minute. Stir in the melted margarine and cool the mixture to room temperature.

3 To make the crêpes, stir all the remaining ingredients except the margarine in a medium-sized bowl until smooth. Cover and refrigerate for 30 minutes.

4 Heat a crêpe pan or small skillet over medium-high heat and brush lightly with some of the margarine. Place 2 tablespoons of the batter in the pan and quickly rotate to spread evenly to the sides. Cook until the batter is no longer shiny, about 30 seconds. Turn the crêpe out onto a clean dish towel and fold into quarters. Repeat with the remaining batter.

5 Lay each crêpe out flat, place 1 teaspoon of the sauce in each crêpe, and roll. Place a dollop of the sauce in the bottom of each dessert plate, place a crêpe on top, and serve.

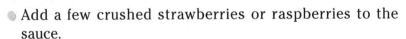

TAKE A CHANCE:

- Add a few crushed strawberries or raspberries to the sauce.

- Garnish with lemon zest.

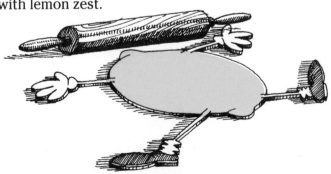

Baked Lemon Soufflé

This recipe just couldn't be easier—even novices will succeed. Put the soufflé in the oven just before you sit down for dinner and enjoy its luscious lemony fragrance throughout the meal.

4 large eggs, separated

grated zest and juice of 1 medium lemon

$\frac{1}{4}$ cup date sugar

Minted Raspberry Sauce (see page 196)

SERVES: 4 · PREPARATION TIME: 45 MINUTES

1 Place the egg yolks in a large bowl and beat with an electric mixer until very thick. Gradually add the lemon zest, lemon juice, and date sugar while continuing to beat the mixture vigorously. Set aside.

2 Place the egg whites in a medium-sized bowl and beat until stiff. Gently fold the egg whites into the lemon mixture. Pour the soufflé mixture into an ungreased 1½-quart soufflé dish. Bake in a 350°F oven for 30 to 35 minutes, or until the soufflé has nearly doubled in size.

3 Spoon into individual dessert dishes and serve warm with the Minted Raspberry Sauce.

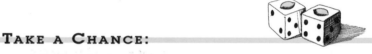

TAKE A CHANCE:

● Pour the mixture into a smaller soufflé dish and add a greased waxed paper "collar" to the dish. Tie the collar on with string and add a piece of tape. The soufflé will rise 2 to 3 inches into the collar. Gently remove the collar before serving.

● Decrease the date sugar by 1 tablespoon and add 1 tablespoon Sweetened Zest (see page 229) to the egg whites.

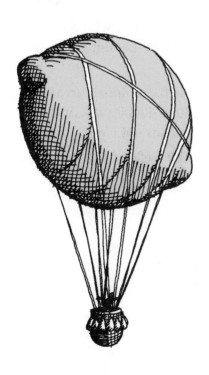

$\mathcal{L}$emon Cupcakes

These cupcakes are a dessert that you can take with you wherever you go.

1¼ cups unbleached white flour

¼ cup malt syrup

1½ teaspoons baking powder

1 large egg

¼ cup light sesame or safflower oil

grated zest of 1 medium lemon

1 teaspoon lemon juice

YIELD: 12 CUPCAKES PREPARATION TIME: 45 MINUTES

1 Place the flour, malt syrup, and baking powder in a large bowl and stir to mix. Place all the remaining ingredients in a small bowl and mix. Slowly add the second mixture to the first and stir to blend.

2 Pour the batter into paper-lined muffin cups, filling them ⅔ full. Bake in a 350°F oven for 20 to 25 minutes, or until a toothpick inserted in the center of a cupcake comes out clean. Immediately remove the muffins from the muffin cups, cool completely, and serve.

Note From a Healthy Lemon:

Use a vegetable-based egg substitute instead of the egg.

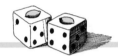

TAKE A CHANCE:

- After the cupcakes have cooled, top them with Sunshine Fresh Lemon Icing (see page 243) or Lemon Cinnamon Glaze (see page 240).

- Make a lemon cake by pouring the batter into a greased 8-inch-square pan and baking for 30 to 40 minutes, or until a toothpick inserted in the center comes out clean.

- If not using paper liners, spray the wells of the muffin tin with a nonstick cooking spray.

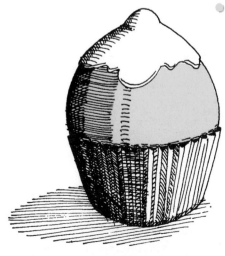

Lemon Cake and Pudding, Too

We never know exactly what to call this lemon-rich dessert treat. During cooking, a rich-tasting cake forms over the top of a delicious, velvety lemon pudding. If you are trying to remove eggs from your diet, this recipe is best skipped. But for those of you who can afford a special treat now and then, give this unique recipe a try!

2 tablespoons safflower oil

$\frac{1}{4}$ cup date sugar

4 large eggs, separated

$\frac{1}{3}$ cup lemon juice

grated zest of 1 medium lemon

3 tablespoons unbleached white flour

1 cup soymilk

SERVES: 4   PREPARATION TIME: 1$\frac{1}{2}$ HOURS

1 Mix the oil and date sugar in a large bowl. Add the egg yolks one at a time, beating well after each addition. Add the lemon juice, lemon zest, and flour, and mix well. Slowly add the soymilk and blend well.

2 Place the egg whites in a small bowl and beat with an electric mixer until stiff. Gently fold the beaten egg whites into the lemon mixture, being careful not to overmix.

3 Pour the batter into a greased 1½-quart casserole dish. Place the casserole dish in a large baking pan containing 1 inch of very hot water and bake in a 350°F oven for 45 to 50 minutes, or until golden. Serve warm or cool.

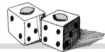

TAKE A CHANCE:

● Top with Fluffy Lemon Topping (see page 242).

● Decrease the date sugar by 1 tablespoon and add 1 tablespoon Sweetened Zest (see page 229) to the egg whites.

Lemonaid

A glass jar or bowl of dried lemon zest will brighten up any room in the house.

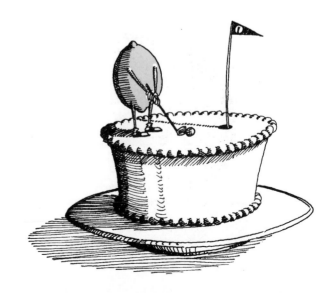

Lemon Angel Cake With Fluffy Lemon Topping

ight as an angel's wings with a creamy, guiltless finish.

1½ cups egg whites
(from 10 to 12 eggs)

1 teaspoon lemon juice

grated zest of 1 medium
lemon

1 cup unbleached white flour

¾ cup Sucanat

Fluffy Lemon Topping
(see page 242)

SERVES: 10   PREPARATION TIME: 1 HOUR

1 Place the egg whites in a large bowl and beat with an electric mixer until foamy. Continue beating until stiff but still moist. Add the lemon juice and lemon zest, and mix just enough to distribute the zest throughout the egg whites.

2 Mix the flour and Sucanat together, and gently fold in the egg whites. Gently pour the batter into an ungreased 10-inch tube pan. Bake in a 375°F oven for 30 to 35 minutes, or until a toothpick inserted in the center comes out clean.

3 Remove the cake from the pan and cool completely. Spread with the Fluffy Lemon Topping and serve.

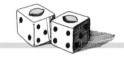

TAKE A CHANCE:

● Use Lemon Cinnamon Glaze (see page 240) instead of the Fluffy Lemon Topping.

● Omit the topping and serve instead with Berry, Berry Lemony (see page 248).

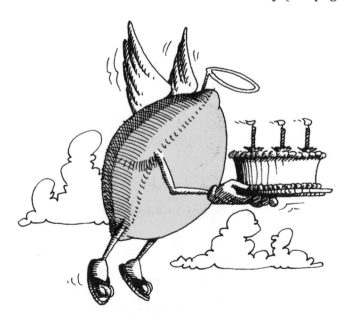

Crunchy Lemon Carrot Cake

We love our carrot cake with everything in it, and this one has everything but the kitchen sink. This cake is very moist because of the pineapple and carrots.

grated zest of 2 medium lemons

1 cup currants

¼ cup chopped walnuts

¼ cup chopped pecans

1 cup whole wheat pastry flour

1 cup unbleached white flour

1½ teaspoons ground cinnamon

½ teaspoon ground nutmeg

½ cup honey

⅓ cup canola oil

1 cup soymilk

½ cup crushed pineapple, drained

1 cup grated carrots

SERVES: 8   PREPARATION TIME: 1 HOUR

1 Place the lemon zest, currants, walnuts, and pecans in a small bowl and mix. Set aside.

2 Place all the remaining ingredients except the pineapple and carrots in a large bowl and mix until well blended. Add the pineapple and stir well. Add the carrots and the currant mixture, and stir well.

3 Pour the batter into a greased and floured 9-x-13-inch baking pan and bake in a 350°F oven for 35 to 45 minutes, or until the cake appears firm but not dry.

4 Cool the cake to room temperature, cut into squares, and serve.

TAKE A CHANCE:

• Top with Lemon Cinnamon Glaze (see page 240) or Sunshine Fresh Lemon Icing (see page 243).

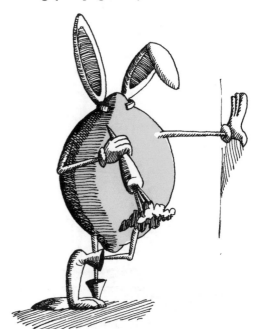

*L*emon-Kissed Pound Cake

here is no such thing as a boring pound cake after it has been kissed by a golden lemon.

grated zest of 2 medium lemons

1 teaspoon lemon juice

⅓ cup soy margarine, at room temperature

1½ cups unbleached white flour

1½ cups whole wheat pastry flour

¼ cup malt powder

½ cup soymilk

1 teaspoon baking powder

2 medium lemons, thinly sliced

S E R V E S : 8   P R E P A R A T I O N   T I M E : 1½ H O U R S

1 Place all the ingredients except the lemon slices in a bowl and stir until well mixed. Pour the batter into a greased bundt pan and bake in a 325°F oven for 1 hour, or until a toothpick inserted in the center comes out clean.

2 Cool the cake in the pan for 10 minutes. Then remove the cake from the pan and cool completely.

3 Arrange the lemon slices along the border of a large serving plate. Place the cake in the center of the plate and serve.

TAKE A CHANCE:

● Sprinkle ground cinnamon on top of the cooled cake.

● Cover the cake with warm Lemon Cinnamon Glaze (see page 240).

● Decorate the plate with lemon-scented geranium leaves.

● Add ½ cup poppy seeds to the batter. Yum! This is Sunny's favorite treat.

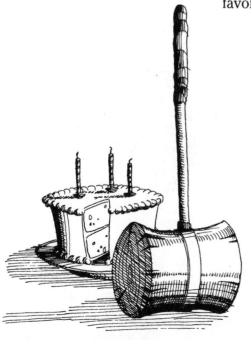

Lemon-Flecked Pie Crust

This pie crust can be used for an 8- or 9-inch pie.

grated zest of 1 medium lemon

1 cup whole wheat pastry flour

¼ cup safflower oil

3 tablespoons hot water

Lemonaid

It only seems like your lemon tree produces 1,000,000 lemons a year. We get about 1,200 from ours. That's still more than 3 lemons a day to enjoy.

YIELD: 1 PIE CRUST   PREPARATION TIME: 20 MINUTES

1 Mix the lemon zest and flour together in a large bowl. Add the oil and stir. The mixture should resemble cornmeal. Sprinkle just enough of the hot water on the mixture, 1 tablespoon at a time, until the flour is moistened and the dough almost cleans the sides of the bowl. Add 1 to 2 more teaspoons of water, if necessary.

2 Shape the dough into a ball and then flatten into a round on a lightly floured board. Using a floured rolling pin, roll the dough 2 inches larger than the pie pan being used. Or, place the dough between two sheets of lightly floured waxed paper and roll it out to size.

3 Fold the dough into quarters and transfer it to the pie pan. If waxed paper is being used, carefully peel off the top sheet of paper. Pick the dough up by the corners of the bottom sheet and place it—paper side up—in the pie pan. Carefully peel off the second sheet.

4 Trim the overhanging dough from the pan and crimp the dough in the pan with your fingers, making a decorative edge. Using a fork, prick the dough on the bottom and sides.

5 To make a prebaked pie crust, bake in a 475°F oven for 8 to 10 minutes, or until golden brown. Otherwise, fill and bake according to the directions given in the recipe you choose.

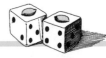

TAKE A CHANCE:

● Make a Citrus-Flecked Pie Crust by mixing grated orange zest with the lemon zest.

● Double the recipe for a two-crust pie.

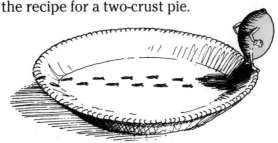

7art Lemon Tartletts

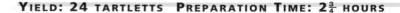

Make enough of these little gems to go around. Two or three bites, and these slices of sunshine are gone. By itself, the lemon curd filling for these tarts can be kept in the refrigerator for 2 weeks or so, but ours almost never lasts that long.

dough for 1 Lemon-Flecked Pie Crust (see page 211)

3 teaspoons date sugar

1 medium egg

2 medium egg whites

3 ounces silken tofu, mashed

grated zest and juice of 3 medium lemons

1 tablespoon soy margarine, melted

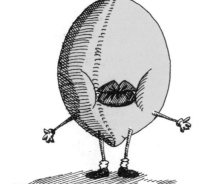

YIELD: 24 TARTLETTS   PREPARATION TIME: 2¾ HOURS

1 Roll out the prepared pie crust dough and cut into two dozen 5-inch rounds. Press the dough pieces into tartlett pans and trim the edges around each pan. Prick the bottoms of the crusts with a fork and bake in a 425°F oven for 8 to 10 minutes, or until lightly golden. Cool completely, then remove the tartlett shells from the pans.

2 Combine the date sugar, egg, and egg whites in the top of a gently simmering double boiler. Using a whisk, beat the mixture until it is frothy, then whip in the tofu. Add the lemon zest, lemon juice, and margarine while continuing to whisk.

3 Bring the water in the bottom of the double boiler to a full boil. Bring the curd mixture to a simmer and stir constantly until the mixture thickens, about 10 minutes. Transfer the curd to a small mixing bowl, cover, and chill until very cold, about 2 hours.

4 Spoon the cooled lemon curd into the baked tartlett shells and serve immediately.

Note From a Healthy Lemon:

To make eggless tartlets, use an amount of egg substitute equivalent to 2 large eggs in place of the egg and egg whites in the recipe. The curd can also be made without the margarine. It will be a bit drier but will still be tasty.

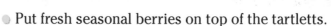

TAKE A CHANCE:

● Put fresh seasonal berries on top of the tartletts.

● Sprinkle additional grated lemon zest over the top of the tartletts, or use a very thin slice of lemon as a garnish.

● Spread the curd by itself on scones, toast, pancakes, or waffles.

The Absolutely Perfect Lemon Meringue Pie

*N*o cookbook on lemons is complete without a recipe for lemon meringue pie. When you're in the mood for the best, try this classic. It's based on the recipe that Sunny's grandmother used to make, but Grandma's recipe never tasted so good!

grated zest and juice of 3 medium lemons

½ cup cold water

3 tablespoons arrowroot

¼ cup plus 2 tablespoons Sucanat

3 large eggs, separated

2 tablespoons soy margarine

1½ cups water, heated almost to boiling

prebaked Lemon-Flecked Pie Crust for 9-inch pie
(see page 211)

¼ teaspoon cream of tartar

SERVES: 8   PREPARATION TIME: 2½ HOURS

1 Combine the lemon juice, cold water, and arrowroot with ¼ cup of the Sucanat in a small saucepan over low heat. Add the egg yolks to the saucepan and stir. Add the margarine and hot water, and bring to a boil, stirring constantly. Reduce the heat to medium and boil for 1 minute. Remove the saucepan from the heat and stir in the lemon zest. Pour the mixture into the prebaked pie crust.

2 Place the egg whites and the cream of tartar in a small bowl and beat with an electric mixer until foamy. Gradually add the remaining 2 tablespoons of Sucanat, beating until stiff peaks form. Place in the pie crust, spreading it over the filling and sealing the edges to prevent shrinking.

3 Bake the pie in a 350°F oven for 12 to 15 minutes, or until the meringue is a delicate brown. Cool for at least 2 hours before serving.

TAKE A CHANCE:

● Sprinkle 2 teaspoons grated lemon zest over the meringue before serving.

● Prepare the meringue with Sweetened Zest (see page 229) instead of the Sucanat.

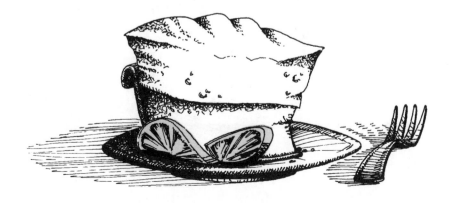

Dreamy Creamy Lemon Pie

We've included this recipe as a special treat. Even made with tofu, this is not for everyday eating, but for an occasional bit of not-too-naughty decadence. You can't beat this pie for creamy texture!

grated zest and juice of 2 medium lemons

2 large egg yolks

$\frac{1}{4}$ cup date sugar

$1\frac{1}{2}$ tablespoons arrowroot

10 ounces silken tofu, drained

prebaked Lemon-Flecked Pie Crust for 8-inch pie (see page 211)

SERVES: 6   PREPARATION TIME: 5 HOURS

1 Place all the ingredients except the tofu and pie crust in the top of a simmering double boiler. Stir constantly until the mixture begins to thicken. Pour the mixture into a small bowl, cover, and refrigerate until cold, about 2 hours.

2 In a medium-sized mixing bowl, beat the tofu with an electric mixer until it's very creamy, then gently fold in the chilled lemon mixture. Spoon the lemon cream into the pastry shell, cover, and refrigerate until set, about 2½ hours. Serve chilled.

TAKE A CHANCE:

● Garnish with Candied Lemon Rosettes (see page 245).

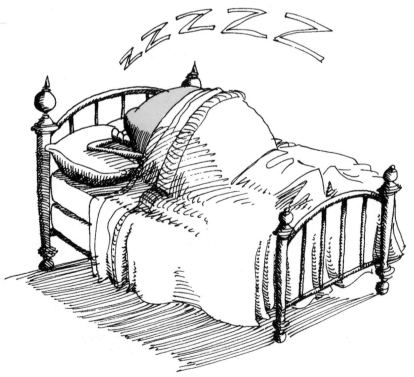

Refreshing Lemon Chiffon Pie

C ool, light, and refreshing chiffon is a special-occasion treat. This recipe is a bit heavy on eggs—so make and serve it with discretion.

---

2 teaspoons agar-agar flakes

$\frac{1}{4}$ cup water

grated zest and juice of 2 medium lemons

4 large eggs, separated

$\frac{1}{4}$ cup malt powder

prebaked Lemon-Flecked Pie Crust for 9-inch pie (see page 211)

SERVES: 6   PREPARATION TIME: 3 HOURS

1 Place the agar-agar and water in the top of a simmering double boiler and stir until the flakes have dissolved. Reduce the heat to medium-low and add all but 1 tablespoon of the lemon zest and all of the lemon juice, egg yolks, and malt powder, mixing well. Stir the mixture constantly until it thickens. Remove the pot from the heat and cool until the mixture begins to set, about 2 hours.

2 Place the egg whites in a medium-sized bowl and beat with an electric mixer until stiff peaks form. Gently fold the egg whites into the lemon mixture. Pour the chiffon into the prebaked pie shell and chill until firm, about 2½ hours.

3 Sprinkle the remaining lemon zest on top of the pie and serve immediately.

TAKE A CHANCE:

○ Decrease the date sugar by 1 tablespoon and add 1 tablespoon Sweetened Zest (see page 229) to the egg whites.

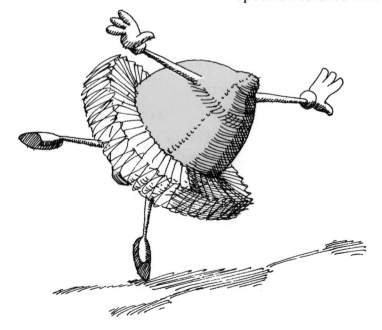

Crusty Lemon Cranberry Pie

This is an especially tart treat that is fun to make, too.

grated zest and juice of 1 medium lemon

$\frac{1}{4}$ cup water

$\frac{1}{4}$ cup concentrated fruit sweetener

1 tablespoon arrowroot

3 cups fresh cranberries

$\frac{1}{2}$ cup currants

$\frac{1}{4}$ cup chopped walnuts

1 teaspoon soy margarine

dough for 2 Lemon-Flecked Pie Crusts (see page 211)

SERVES: 6   PREPARATION TIME: 2 HOURS

1 Place the lemon zest, lemon juice, water, concentrated fruit sweetener, and arrowroot in a medium-sized saucepan and stir to mix. Heat to boiling over high heat, stirring constantly.

2 Reduce the heat to low and add the cranberries, currants, and walnuts. Simmer for 5 minutes, stirring constantly. Remove the pan from the heat and stir in the margarine. Cool.

3 Roll out half the pie crust dough to 11 inches. Fit the crust into a 9-inch pie plate, leaving the excess pastry hanging over the side of the plate. Pour the cooled filling into the crust.

4 Roll out the other half of the pie crust dough to 11 inches and place it over the filling. Trim the crusts, pinching the edges together.

5 Using a sharp knife, make several short slashes in the top crust. Bake the pie in a 425°F oven for 35 to 40 minutes, or until the crust turns golden brown. Cool to room temperature before serving.

TAKE A CHANCE:

● Use raisins instead of the currants.

● Add a dash of ground cinnamon to the cranberries.

● Use frozen cranberries instead of the fresh. (You need not thaw the berries before using them.)

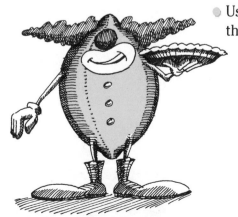

Chapter 10

Dressings, Sauces, and Toppings— Lemon Miracles

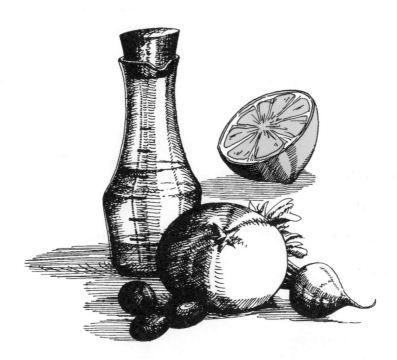

Even if your recipe already contains lemon—and especially if it doesn't—chances are that the lemony miracles in this chapter can enhance and enliven the flavor of the finished dish. You'll find something in this chapter to go with almost any food you make. Some of the toppings are sweet. Others are tart. Others offer new tangy taste sensations. All are lemony and delightful.

*L*emon Honey Vinaigrette

A slightly sweet dressing that goes well with your favorite fruit or vegetable salads.

juice of 1 medium lemon

2 tablespoons extra virgin olive oil

1 tablespoon red wine vinegar

2 tablespoons honey

½ teaspoon dry mustard

YIELD: ½ CUP   PREPARATION TIME: 10 MINUTES

1 Combine all the ingredients in a glass jar, cover, and shake until thoroughly mixed.

2 Use immediately, or cover the dressing and refrigerate until it is needed.

TAKE A CHANCE:

● Add ½ teaspoon cayenne pepper or paprika to the honey, and let it sit for 30 minutes before mixing the dressing.

● Add the grated zest of 1 lemon.

● Add ½ teaspoon chopped fresh basil or oregano.

Lemonaid

When a recipe calls for wine or vinegar, substitute lemon juice for a brighter taste.

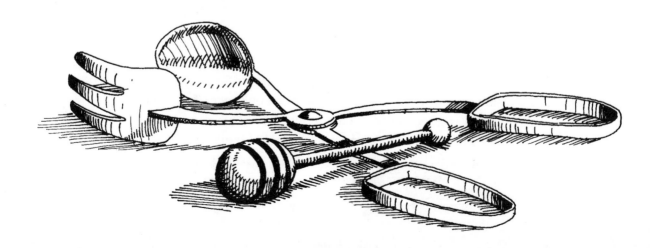

Lemon Poppy Seed Dressing

Don't limit your love for lemon and poppy seeds to muffins. This delightful dressing is particularly refreshing when served over a fruit salad, and it is terrific on veggies.

---

grated zest and juice of 1 medium lemon

2 tablespoons light sesame or safflower oil

$\frac{1}{2}$ teaspoon dry mustard

1 teaspoon date sugar

1 tablespoon poppy seeds

YIELD: $\frac{1}{4}$ CUP PREPARATION TIME: 30 MINUTES

1 Combine all the ingredients except the poppy seeds in a glass jar, cover, and shake. Add the poppy seeds and shake until thoroughly mixed. Refrigerate for 20 minutes.

2 Use immediately, or cover the dressing and refrigerate until it is needed.

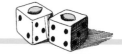

TAKE A CHANCE:

- Add 1 teaspoon finely minced onion.
- Use honey instead of the date sugar.

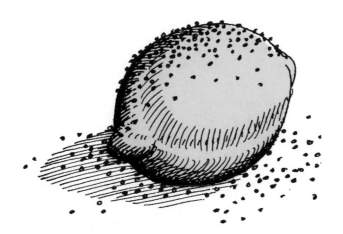

Spicy Southwest Lemon Dressing

Here is a salad dressing for the more adventurous. Try this with sliced avocados and tomatoes, sprinkled with walnuts.

juice of 1 medium lemon

1 small red or green jalapeño pepper, finely minced

1 teaspoon minced fresh cilantro

2 tablespoons extra virgin olive oil

$\frac{1}{4}$ teaspoon chili powder

YIELD: $\frac{1}{4}$ CUP   PREPARATION TIME: 10 MINUTES

1 Combine all the ingredients in a glass jar, cover, and shake until thoroughly mixed.

2 Use immediately, or cover the dressing and refrigerate until it is needed.

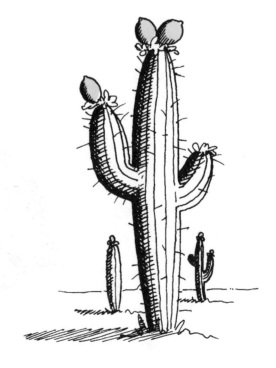

TAKE A CHANCE:

● Use cayenne pepper or paprika instead of the chili powder.

● Omit the jalapeño pepper and add 1 teaspoon diced onion or shallot.

Lemonaid

A diluted lemon juice rinse will help you to eliminate that bothersome case of dandruff. Just work it in and rinse with cool water.

*L*ight Lemon Vinaigrette

This vinaigrette gives salad a cool lemon taste. There is nothing more simple or delicious. Change the herb used depending on the season and the salad.

juice of 1 medium lemon

1 large garlic clove, finely minced

2 tablespoons light sesame or safflower oil

1 tablespoon balsamic vinegar

1 teaspoon dried oregano

$\frac{1}{4}$ teaspoon freshly ground black pepper

YIELD: $\frac{1}{4}$ CUP   PREPARATION TIME: 30 MINUTES

1 Combine all the ingredients in a glass jar, cover, and shake until well blended. Let sit for 20 minutes.

2 Use immediately, or cover and refrigerate for up to 2 days.

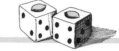

TAKE A CHANCE:

● Make the dressing with olive oil.

● Add 2 tablespoons Dijon mustard to the recipe for Lemon Dijon Vinaigrette. Use this for heartier salads, such as Zesty Tofu With Pasta and Peas (see page 81).

● Add 1 tablespoon mashed silken tofu for a creamy texture.

● Use the vinaigrette as a marinade.

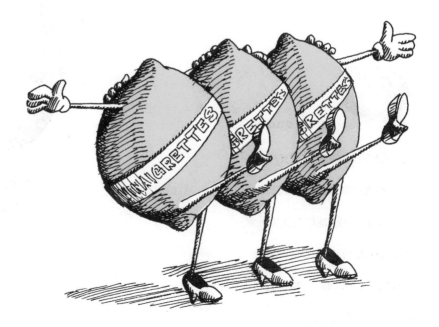

*F*eta Cheese Dressing

By crumbling up the cheese and tossing it in the dressing, you'll get a rich creamy texture enhanced by a few drops of liquid gold.

juice of 1 medium lemon

1 large garlic clove, finely minced

½ teaspoon dried oregano

3 tablespoons extra virgin olive oil

3 tablespoons crumbled feta cheese

YIELD: ¼ CUP   PREPARATION TIME: 20 MINUTES

1 Combine all the ingredients except the feta cheese in a small bowl and mix well. Add the cheese and mix again. Let the dressing sit for 10 minutes.

2 Immediately add the dressing to a salad, toss, and serve.

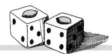

TAKE A CHANCE:

○ Use fresh oregano instead of the dried.

○ Use basil instead of the oregano.

○ Experiment with different types of feta cheese and olive oil for different tastes.

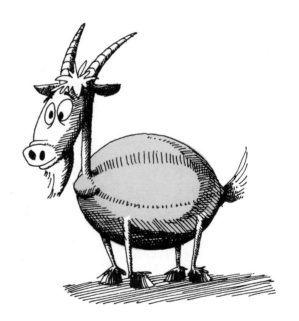

Lemonaid

Create a refreshing pore-tightening facial mask by mashing cucumbers and almond meal together with lemon juice.

Tart Citrus Vinaigrette

This tart fruit taste goes well on a mixture of bibb lettuce, red leaf lettuce, and radicchio.

2 tablespoons lemon juice

3 tablespoons orange juice

2 tablespoons extra virgin olive oil

1 tablespoon raspberry vinegar

$\frac{1}{4}$ teaspoon freshly ground black pepper

YIELD: $\frac{1}{2}$ CUP   PREPARATION TIME: 20 MINUTES

1 Combine all the ingredients in a glass jar, cover, and shake until well mixed. Let sit for 10 minutes.

2 Use immediately, or cover and refrigerate for up to 2 days.

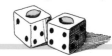

TAKE A CHANCE:

- Warm the vinaigrette slightly before pouring it over the greens.

- Warm and serve over pasta.

- Add ¼ teaspoon grated lemon or orange zest to the vinaigrette.

- Substitute blueberry vinegar for the raspberry vinegar.

Lemonaid

Mix and store salad dressing in glass jars. The dressing will stay fresher, and the acidity of the lemon won't cause the dressing to take on a plastic flavor.

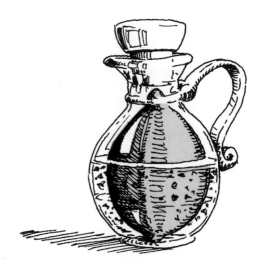

Cooked Lemony Citrus Dressing

A lemony, low-cal alternative to French dressing.

- ¼ cup Lemon-Touched Ketchup (see page 239)
- ¼ cup lemon juice
- ½ cup orange juice
- 1 tablespoon light sesame or safflower oil
- 1 teaspoon arrowroot
- ¼ teaspoon date sugar
- ¼ teaspoon paprika
- ¼ teaspoon dry mustard
- ¼ teaspoon hot sauce

YIELD: ¾ CUP   PREPARATION TIME: 1 HOUR

1 Combine all the ingredients in a small saucepan and bring to a boil over high heat. Reduce the heat to low and simmer the mixture for 1 minute, stirring constantly. Transfer the dressing to a glass jar, cover, and refrigerate for 1 hour, or until chilled.

2 Use immediately, or cover the dressing and refrigerate until it is needed.

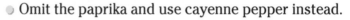

TAKE A CHANCE:

- Omit the paprika and use cayenne pepper instead.
- Use regular ketchup instead of the homemade Lemon-Touched Ketchup.

Lemonaid

Used on your hair, a lemon juice rinse counteracts the alkalinity of commercial shampoos, stripping away the buildup.

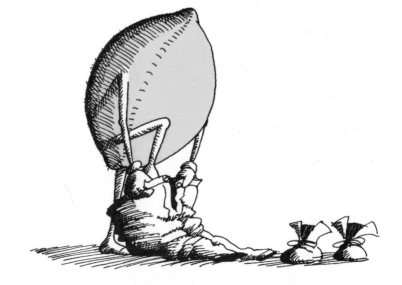

Lemon Garlic Croutons

What could be better with your soup or salad? We certainly can't think of anything!

3 slices stale sourdough bread, cut into ½-inch cubes

2 tablespoons soy margarine

1 large garlic clove, coarsely chopped

grated zest and juice of 1 medium lemon

YIELD: 1 CUP   PREPARATION TIME: 30 MINUTES

1 Place the bread cubes on a cookie sheet and bake in a 250°F oven for 15 minutes, turning once. The cubes should be well dried and just lightly browned. Set aside.

2 Melt the margarine in a large skillet. Add the garlic and sauté lightly for 1 minute, or until you can smell the garlic strongly. Do not let the garlic brown or it will become bitter. Using a slotted spoon, remove the garlic.

3 Add the lemon zest and the lemon juice to the skillet and stir. Add the toasted bread cubes and stir gently until the cubes have absorbed all of the margarine.

4 Cool the croutons and use immediately in soups or salads.

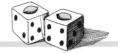

TAKE A CHANCE:

○ Add a small amount of snipped fresh dill to the pan along with the lemon.

○ Increase the amount of grated lemon zest.

○ Use lemon thyme or lemon balm instead of the grated lemon zest.

○ Use whole wheat or multigrain bread.

Lemonaid

When making potpourri, add the dried flowers and leaves of a lemon tree to the mix for a different twist. Add some dried cranberries and orange slices for a dash of color.

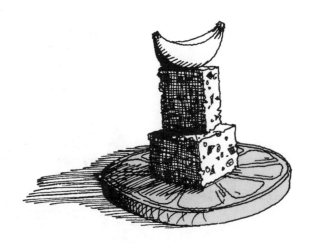

Lemongrass Vinegar

*F*lavored vinegars are very easy to make and really perk up dull dressings, marinades, and sauces. Experiment!

1 large stalk fresh lemongrass

1 cup rice vinegar

YIELD: 1 CUP   PREPARATION TIME: 4 DAYS

1 Using a sharp knife, thinly slice the bottom 8 inches of the lemongrass stalk. Using the side of the knife, lightly bruise the slices to release the flavor of the lemongrass.

2 Place the slices in a glass jar and add the vinegar. Cover with a lid and steep in a cool dark place for 4 days to 2 weeks, depending on the strength desired.

3 Strain the vinegar into another jar and discard the lemongrass. Seal and store at room temperature for up to 6 months, adding to recipes—including salad dressings—as your imagination inspires.

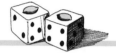

TAKE A CHANCE:

● Add a few flakes of crushed red pepper during the steeping process.

● Make vinegars using lemon basil and lemon balm instead of the lemongrass.

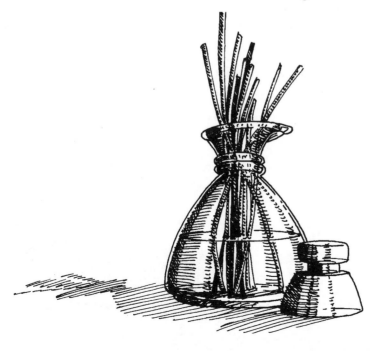

Lemon Pepper

Get in the habit of grating the zest of every lemon before squeezing. If the recipe doesn't call for the zest, just dry it out and add pepper. Don't make this in huge quantities. Like other spices, pepper begins to lose its potency after six months.

grated zest of 3 medium lemons

$\frac{1}{4}$ cup freshly ground black pepper

YIELD: $\frac{1}{4}$ CUP   PREPARATION TIME: 2 DAYS

1 Spread the lemon zest on paper toweling and let it dry at room temperature for 48 hours.

2 Transfer to a small glass jar, add the pepper, cover, and shake until thoroughly mixed. Store at room temperature for up to 6 months.

TAKE A CHANCE:

- Grind a combination of peppercorns—black, green, white, and pink. (We recommend using this combination every time you grind pepper. Each peppercorn has its own flavor. When eating a dish enhanced by this mixture, every forkful will have a slightly different taste.)

- Add you own dried herbs, such as parsley, cilantro, and oregano, to make Lemon Herb Pepper. (Don't use dried parsley from a store—for anything!)

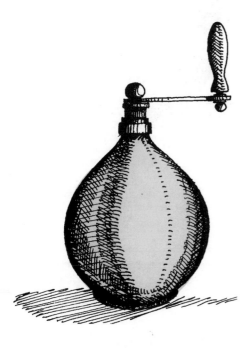

Gremolata

We keep fresh Gremolata on the table to use as salt. It's great on rice and other grains, and adds a bit of spice to ordinary steamed vegetables.

2 tablespoons finely chopped lemon zest

2 medium garlic cloves, finely chopped

2 tablespoons finely chopped fresh parsley

YIELD: ¼ CUP   PREPARATION TIME: 5 MINUTES

1 Toss all the ingredients with a fork in a small cup.

2 Serve fresh in a small bowl. Just sprinkle the Gremolata on any dish you feel needs a little zest.

TAKE A CHANCE:

- Adjust the amounts of the lemon and garlic for different tastes.

- Add crushed red pepper to spice up the mixture.

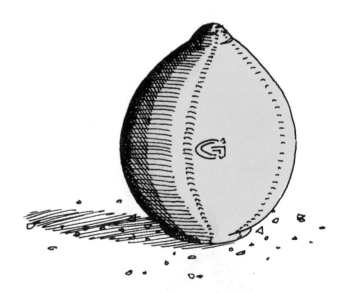

Lemonaid

Always grate the lemon zest before you juice the lemon.

Sweetened Zest

Used sparingly, this easy-to-make flavoring is a treat in coffee, tea, cereal, cookies, cakes, muffins, or anything else that needs a bit of lemony sweetness.

grated zest of 2 medium lemons

½ cup Sucanat

YIELD: ½ CUP   PREPARATION TIME: 2 HOURS

1 Spread the grated lemon zest on paper toweling. Dry at room temperature for 1 hour, turning occasionally.

2 Mix the zest thoroughly with the Sucanat and place in a small, tightly covered glass jar. Let sit for at least 1 hour before using.

3 Mix thoroughly before using. Sweetened Zest will keep for several weeks.

TAKE A CHANCE:

- Add orange zest for Citrus Sugar.

Lemonaid

Napkins or washcloths rinsed in equal parts of warm water and lemon juice will clean grease from your hands after dinner.

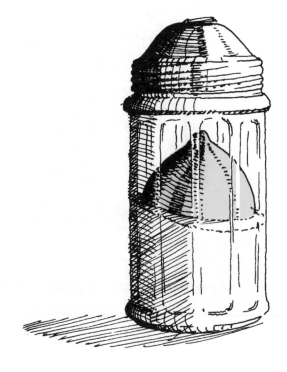

Lemony Hollandaise Sauce

Delicate, creamy, and oh so lemony! Try this sauce over steamed fresh asparagus.

¼ cup lemon juice

2 large egg yolks

5 tablespoons safflower oil

pinch of cayenne pepper

YIELD: ½ CUP   PREPARATION TIME: 10 MINUTES

1 Place the lemon juice and egg yolks in a small saucepan and mix over low heat until smooth. Gradually add the oil, stirring constantly. Add the cayenne pepper and continue stirring until the sauce thickens.

2 Spoon the warm sauce over steamed vegetables and serve immediately.

Note From a Healthy Lemon:

Use a vegetable-based egg substitute instead of the egg yolks.

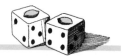

TAKE A CHANCE:

● Stir in 1 teaspoon grated lemon zest before serving.

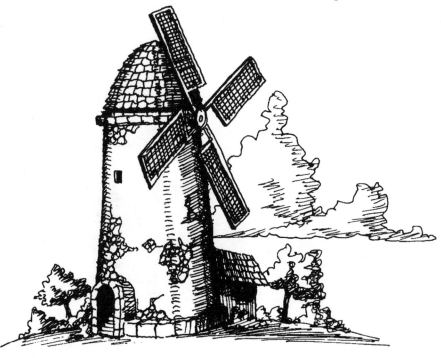

Lemon Vegetable Sauce

All vegetables should be lucky enough to lie beneath a blanket of this lovely sauce.

½ cup Lemon Vegetable Broth (see page 86)

2 teaspoons minced onion

1 large garlic clove, finely chopped

juice of ½ medium lemon

½ teaspoon arrowroot

¼ teaspoon freshly ground black pepper

YIELD: ½ CUP   PREPARATION TIME: 10 MINUTES

1 Heat 2 tablespoons of the broth in a small saucepan over medium heat and sauté the onion and garlic for 1 minute. Add the lemon juice and the remaining broth, and simmer for 1 minute. Add the arrowroot and stir until the sauce thickens. Add the pepper and stir.

2 Serve hot over broccoli, cauliflower, carrots, or almost any other vegetable.

TAKE A CHANCE:

- Add 1 teaspoon dried sage or thyme.
- Add ½ teaspoon grated lemon zest.

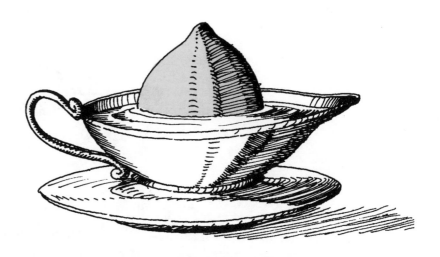

Zesty Barbecue Sauce

Try this zesty barbecue sauce on Grilled Tofu (see page 118) or Lemon-Kissed Soy Burgers (see page 127), and make sure there is enough to pass around the dinner table!

1 cup Spicy Lemon Ketchup (see page 238)

juice of 1 medium lemon

1 lemon slice cut $\frac{1}{2}$-inch thick

1 large garlic clove, quartered

1 teaspoon dry mustard

1 teaspoon chili powder

1 teaspoon Worcestershire sauce

$\frac{1}{2}$ teaspoon dried thyme

$\frac{1}{2}$ teaspoon dried sage

1 bay leaf

$\frac{1}{4}$ teaspoon freshly ground black pepper

YIELD: 1 CUP PREPARATION TIME: 1$\frac{1}{4}$ HOURS

1 Mix all the ingredients in a medium-sized bowl. Cover and let sit at room temperature for 1 hour.

2 Discard the lemon slice and bay leaf, and use the sauce immediately by brushing onto grilled foods just before they are finished cooking. If any sauce remains, transfer to a glass jar, cover, and refrigerate for up to 3 days.

TAKE A CHANCE:

● Omit the chili powder.

● Add or subtract herbs, depending on your taste.

● Use Lemon-Touched Ketchup (see page 239) instead of the Spicy Lemon Ketchup.

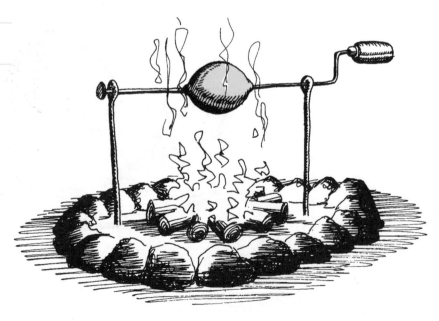

Zippy Cocktail Sauce

Your taste buds will know for certain that this is the best cocktail sauce ever made. It's so easy to make, you'll never use store-bought cocktail sauce again.

juice of ½ medium lemon

1 cup Spicy Lemon Ketchup (see page 238)

¼ cup prepared white horse-radish

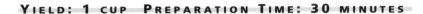

1 Mix all the ingredients in a medium-sized bowl. Cover and refrigerate for at least 30 minutes.

2 Serve cold, or cover tightly and refrigerate until it is needed.

TAKE A CHANCE:

- Turn up the heat by adding more horseradish.
- Make your own horseradish instead of using a prepared sauce.
- Add 1 teaspoon grated lemon zest.
- Add 1 teaspoon Worcestershire sauce.

Lemonaid

Keep an unwrapped lemon half in the back of your refrigerator to eliminate bad odors.

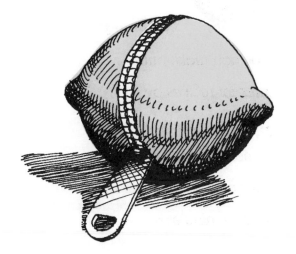

Almost Sour Cream

Try this on your next baked potato instead of the usual fat-laden sour cream. You almost won't know the difference. This can be used as a substitute for sour cream in most recipes.

juice of ½ medium lemon

1 cup nonfat cottage cheese

2 tablespoons tofu mayonnaise or natural mayonnaise (optional)

YIELD: 1 CUP   PREPARATION TIME: 5 MINUTES

1 Place the lemon juice, cottage cheese, and mayonnaise in a blender or food processor, and pulse until smooth.

2 Serve immediately, or cover and refrigerate for up to 2 days.

TAKE A CHANCE:

- Add 1 teaspoon grated lemon zest.
- Use ½ cup nonfat cottage cheese and ½ cup mashed silken tofu.
- Add some chopped fresh herbs, such as dill or oregano.
- Serve as a dip for fresh vegetables or as a spread on whole wheat crackers.

Lemonaid

You can make buttermilk for recipes by adding 1 tablespoon lemon juice to 1 cup milk and letting it sit for five minutes.

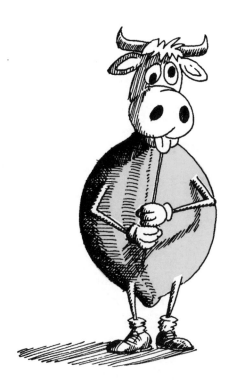

Mock Lemon Butter

There is nothing that more quickly and easily enhances the flavor of almost any dish than a simple lemon butter. This version uses soy margarine in place of high-cholesterol butter.

---

grated zest and juice of 1 medium lemon

½ cup soy margarine, at room temperature

Lemonaid

Lemon juice can be added to a dish that has been oversalted to help minimize the salty taste.

YIELD: ½ CUP   PREPARATION TIME: 30 MINUTES

1 Place the lemon zest, lemon juice, and margarine in a small bowl and beat vigorously with a spoon until the ingredients are well blended.

2 Cover the butter and let it sit for 30 minutes at room temperature, to allow the flavors to develop. Use immediately, or place in a serving dish or mold and refrigerate for up to 4 days. (The longer the mixture has a chance to sit before being used, the more intense the lemon flavor will be.)

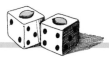

TAKE A CHANCE:

● Omit the lemon juice and zest, and use lemon balm or lemon verbena instead.

● Make Herbed Mock Lemon Butter by adding ½ teaspoon of a fresh herb such as oregano, mint, basil, dill, or sage. If using dried herbs, first soak them in 1 teaspoon lemon juice for 15 minutes. This will bring out their flavor.

● Make a spicy butter by adding ½ teaspoon crushed garlic, paprika, minced onion, chili powder, or cayenne pepper.

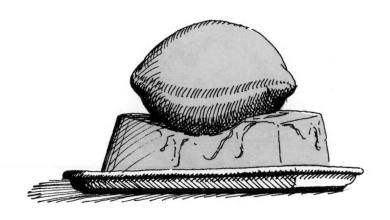

Lemony Yogurt Cheese Spread

his lemony spread is made from nonfat plain yogurt and can be used like cream cheese on breads and crackers.

4 cups plain nonfat yogurt

grated zest of 1 medium lemon

YIELD: 1½ CUPS   PREPARATION TIME: 12 HOURS

1 Pour the yogurt in a yogurt strainer, or in a colander lined with a double thickness of cheesecloth and set over a large bowl. Cover with plastic wrap and refrigerate overnight.

2 Discard the yogurt liquid and mix the remaining yogurt cheese with the lemon zest. Serve immediately, or transfer to a glass jar, cover, and refrigerate for up to 1 week.

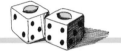

TAKE A CHANCE:

- Use lemon yogurt instead of the plain yogurt.
- Depending on your preferences, mix the yogurt cheese with lemon pepper, lemon balm, or lemon mint instead of the lemon zest.
- Add 1 teaspoon mashed strawberries.

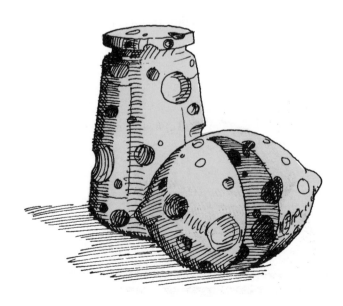

Lemon Mayonnaise

This is a thick and creamy mayonnaise with a touch of lemon.

3 tablespoons lemon juice

1 large egg

$\frac{1}{8}$ teaspoon freshly ground white pepper

1 teaspoon dry mustard

5 tablespoons light sesame or safflower oil

YIELD: $\frac{1}{2}$ CUP   PREPARATION TIME: 5 MINUTES

1 Place the lemon juice, egg, and pepper in a blender or food processor, and blend until smooth. Add the dry mustard and blend to mix. With the motor running, add the oil in a very slow stream until the mixture becomes creamy.

2 Use the mayonnaise immediately, or transfer to a glass jar, cover, and refrigerate for up to 2 days.

Note From a Healthy Lemon:

Use a vegetable-based egg substitute instead of the egg.

TAKE A CHANCE:

- Add ½ teaspoon dried oregano with the white pepper.
- Use half light sesame oil and half olive oil.

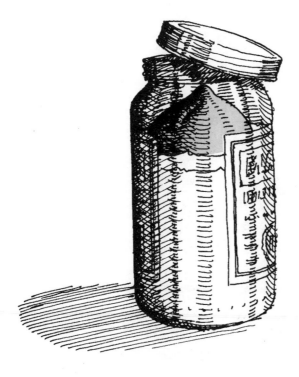

Spicy Lemon Ketchup

This ketchup is zestier than regular ketchup and lacks the preservatives and extra sugar of the commercial variety.

grated zest of 1 medium lemon

½ cup lemon juice

12 ounces tomato paste

½ cup water

1 teaspoon dried oregano

½ teaspoon ground cumin

⅛ teaspoon ground nutmeg

⅛ teaspoon freshly ground black pepper

½ teaspoon dry mustard

1 medium garlic clove, crushed

YIELD: 1¾ CUPS   PREPARATION TIME: 15 MINUTES

1 Place all the ingredients in a medium-sized bowl and mix thoroughly.

2 Use the ketchup immediately, or transfer to a glass jar, cover, and refrigerate for up to 1 week.

TAKE A CHANCE:

- Omit the lemon juice and zest, and use cider vinegar to make a more conventional ketchup.

- Make a spicier ketchup by adding ½ teaspoon crushed garlic, paprika, finely minced onion, chili powder, or cayenne pepper.

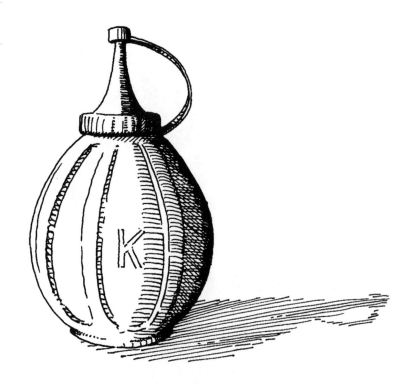

Lemon-Touched Ketchup

T his is a less lemony, less spicy ketchup than Spicy Lemon Ketchup (see page 238). It doesn't take very long to make, and it's much better than anything you can buy!

1 tablespoon lemon juice

2 cups tomato purée

1 cup light sesame or safflower oil

2 tablespoons date sugar

2 tablespoons white vinegar

$\frac{1}{8}$ teaspoon shoyu or tamari sauce

YIELD: 3 CUPS PREPARATION TIME: 20 MINUTES

1 Place all the ingredients in a medium-sized saucepan, stir to blend, and cook for 5 minutes over low heat, stirring frequently. Adjust the ingredients to taste.

2 Cool to room temperature and use immediately, or transfer to a glass jar, cover, and refrigerate for up to 1week.

TAKE A CHANCE:

● Add 2 tablespoons puréed onion.

● Go wild and add 1 teaspoon puréed jalapeño pepper.

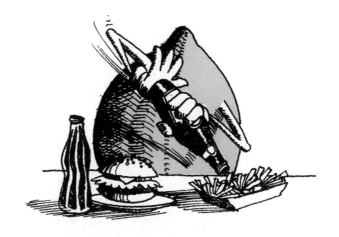

Lemonaid

Lemons on the tree take 7 to 8 months to ripen.

*L*emon Cinnamon Glaze

This glaze, made tart and tasty with citrus and rich with cinnamon, will add a lemony spice to cakes and tea breads.

grated zest and juice of 1 medium lemon

$\frac{1}{4}$ cup concentrated fruit sweetener

6 tablespoons water

$\frac{1}{2}$ teaspoon ground cinnamon

$\frac{1}{8}$ teaspoon ground cloves

YIELD: $\frac{1}{4}$ CUP   PREPARATION TIME: 20 MINUTES

1 Place all the ingredients in a small saucepan, stir to blend, and simmer over low heat for 15 minutes.

2 Pour the hot glaze over cakes, cupcakes, or breads immediately before serving.

TAKE A CHANCE:

● Substitute 1 cinnamon stick for the ground spice and remove the stick before using the glaze.

● Add ⅛ teaspoon allspice.

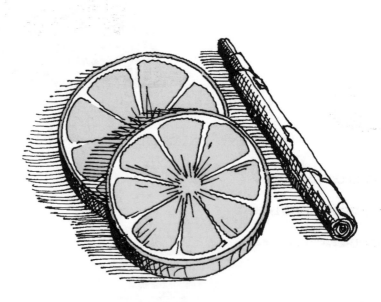

Honey and Lemon Spread

This luscious spread is destined to become a pantry staple. Easy to make, it's great on toast, pancakes, or waffles, or as a marinade for chicken or tofu.

juice of 3 medium lemons
(reserve 1 lemon hull)

½ cup honey

YIELD: ¾ CUP   PREPARATION TIME: 2 HOURS

1 Place the lemon juice and honey in an airtight glass jar. Cut the dimpled end off the reserved lemon hull and cut the hull into strips. Add to the honey and stir. The honey will be thin. Cover and let sit at room temperature for 2 hours.

2 Remove the lemon strips from the jar. Use the spread immediately, or cover and store at room temperature for up to 1 week.

TAKE A CHANCE:

- Add 1 teaspoon chili powder or cayenne pepper.
- Use a flavored honey, such as mesquite or wildflower.
- If using the spread as a marinade—or if you just want more lemon flavor—place several slices of whole lemon in the honey.

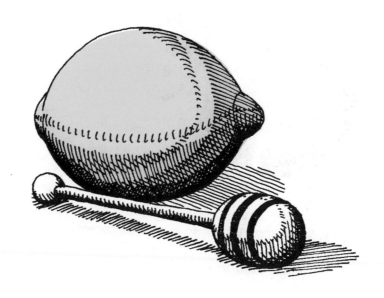

Fluffy Lemon Topping

This is a topping that can also be served on its own as a luscious lemon mousse.

grated zest of 1 medium lemon

1 tablespoon lemon juice

$10\frac{1}{2}$ ounces extra-firm silken tofu

$\frac{1}{4}$ cup mild honey

1 teaspoon vanilla extract

YIELD: $1\frac{1}{2}$ CUPS PREPARATION TIME: $1\frac{1}{4}$ HOURS

1 Place all the ingredients in a blender or food processor, and blend until smooth and creamy, scraping the sides of the container occasionally. Transfer to a small bowl, cover, and chill for at least 1 hour.

2 Serve cold, spooning or drizzling the topping over cake.

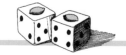

TAKE A CHANCE:

● Add more vanilla and decrease the amount of lemon.

● Use half honey and half concentrated fruit sweetener.

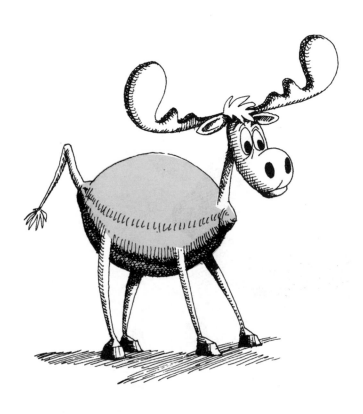

Sunshine Fresh Lemon Icing

Smooth, gooey, and lemony fresh for those times when you just have to have an icing. It's like a lemon caramel.

¼ cup tahini

¼ cup soymilk

¼ cup malt syrup

grated zest and juice of 1 medium lemon

YIELD: ¾ CUP   PREPARATION TIME: 15 MINUTES

1 Mix the tahini and the soymilk in a small bowl. Add the malt syrup and mix again.

2 Add the lemon zest and lemon juice to the soymilk mixture and stir until smooth. Add additional lemon juice to bring the icing to the desired spreading consistency.

3 Spread over cooled cakes, cupcakes, or tea breads.

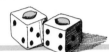

TAKE A CHANCE:

• Add the grated zest of 1 orange.

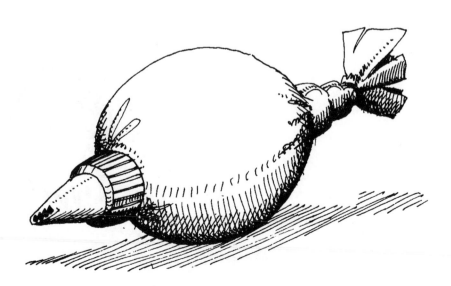

Lemon Fruit Syrup

This concentrated syrup is great to have on hand for almost any occasion. Use it in Citrus Slushies (see page 38), in place of maple syrup on pancakes and waffles, or instead of margarine on your morning scone.

juice of 2 medium lemons

1 pint strawberries, hulled and cut in half

2 teaspoons concentrated fruit sweetener

2 tablespoons mild honey

$\frac{1}{2}$ cup water

YIELD: 2 CUPS   PREPARATION TIME: 45 MINUTES

1 Place all the ingredients in a small saucepan and bring to a boil over high heat. Reduce the heat to low and cook for 30 minutes, stirring occasionally, until the liquid becomes a thin syrup.

2 Place two layers of cheesecloth in a sieve and strain the syrup, using a wooden spoon to push out as much liquid as possible from the berries. Pour the remaining syrup into a glass jar, cover, and cool.

3 Use the syrup immediately, or cover and refrigerate for up to 1 week.

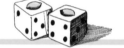

TAKE A CHANCE:

- Use raspberries or blueberries instead of the strawberries.
- If fresh fruit is not available, use 2 packages of frozen berries.

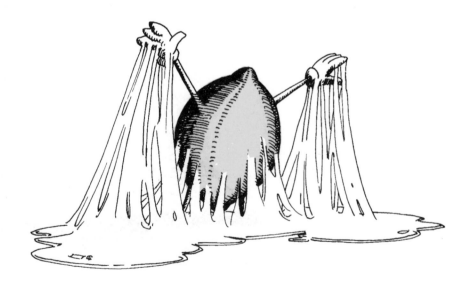

Candied Lemon Rosettes

These rosettes are not meant to be eaten, but are easy to make and use as a colorful garnish for anything.

$\frac{1}{3}$ cup water

$\frac{1}{2}$ cup date sugar

zest of 2 medium lemons, each cut in one continuous strip

4 fresh mint leaves

1 cherry, pitted and halved

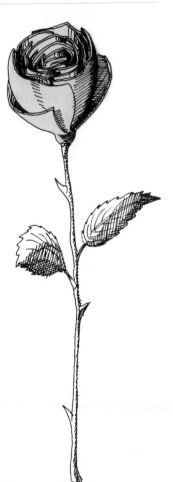

YIELD: 2 ROSETTES   PREPARATION TIME: 20 MINUTES

1 Place the water in a small saucepan and bring to a boil over high heat. Add the date sugar and stir constantly until the sugar is dissolved. Reduce the heat to low, add the lemon zest, and simmer for 10 minutes. Using a fork or a slotted spoon, remove the zest, place on waxed paper, and allow to cool.

2 Place the mint leaves on the surface to be decorated, using 2 leaves for each rosette. Spiral the candied peels to form a decorative rosette over the leaves. Place a cherry half in the center of each spiral.

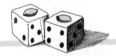

TAKE A CHANCE:

- To make a more colorful garnish, use both a lemon and an orange zest.

- Cut a large mint or basil leaf into a long strip and roll to form the stem of a flower.

- Having a hard time making a continuous zest? Make the zest as long as possible and candy as described above. Then form several smaller flowers with the shorter peels.

Moroccan Preserved Lemons

U sed often in Moroccan cooking, these salty-sour preserved lemons will keep for up to one year.

4 medium lemons, at room temperature

$\frac{1}{4}$ cup sea salt

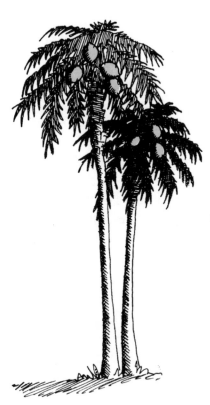

YIELD: 1 QUART   PREPARATION TIME: 30 DAYS

1 Cut each lemon in quarters from the top to within ½ inch of the bottom. Do not separate the quarters. Sprinkle the flesh with half the salt and press the quarters back into place.

2 Place 1 tablespoon of the salt on the bottom of a 1-quart glass jar. Tightly pack the lemons into the jar, adding salt to each layer as you add more lemons. As you push them down, the lemons will release their juices. When you're done, lemon juice should completely cover the fruit. If it doesn't, fill the jar with more fresh-squeezed lemon juice.

3 Seal the jar and store for 30 days at room temperature, shaking the jar each day.

4 Rinse the lemons under running water before using. (Don't worry about any white film seen on some lemons. It's harmless.) Lemon quarters can be used with or without the pulp and don't need to be refrigerated after opening.

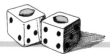

TAKE A CHANCE:

- Spice up your preserved lemons by adding a cinnamon stick, a bay leaf, or a few peppercorns to the layers of lemons.

- Use the lemon pulp or the zest to add a piquant taste to salad dressings or to A Very Tart Virgin Mary (see page 41).

- If you can't wait for 30 days, cut the lemons in the manner described above and arrange them in a baking dish just large enough to hold them in one layer. Pour salt and lemon juice over the lemons, completely covering them. Cover with aluminum foil and bake in a 200°F oven for 3 hours, stirring occasionally. Cool the lemons and brine, and place in an airtight jar. The taste will be slightly different, but the lemons will still be wonderful.

Chapter 11

Breakfast—
Under the Lemon Tree

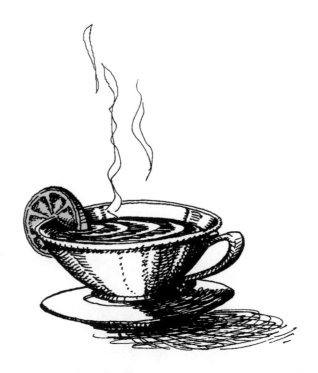

on't leave the lemon far from the breakfast table. Its tart, refreshing taste will add a bounce to your step and start you dreaming of ways to get more lemon freshness and goodness all day long.

Berry, Berry Lemony

A delicious lemony morning eye opener—or a lunch, snack, or dinner treat. Can you think of a better way to get all your fruit each day? If you're always on the run, prepare everything the night before.

grated zest and juice of 2 medium lemons

1 cup strawberries, hulled and cut in half

1 cup blueberries

1 cup raspberries

1 cup blackberries

4 fresh mint leaves

YIELD: 4 CUPS   PREPARATION TIME: 1 HOUR

1 Place the lemon zest, lemon juice, and berries in a medium-sized bowl and mix. Cover and refrigerate for 1 hour.

2 Transfer the berries to individual serving dishes, garnish with the mint, and serve.

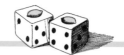

TAKE A CHANCE:

● Add coconut to the berries.

● Add sunflower seeds or chopped walnuts before serving.

● Add bananas, apples, or grapes.

● Instead of using the berries, use chunks of papaya and mango.

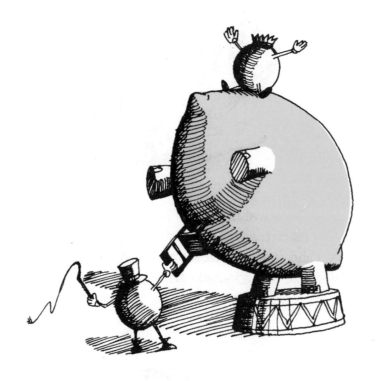

Morning Melon

It's not always necessary to create melon balls or melon baskets. Just dress up your morning melon a little.

1 large melon such as cantaloupe or honeydew

1 cup Lemony Yogurt Cheese Spread (see page 236)

½ cup blueberries

¼ cup chopped walnuts

SERVES: 4   PREPARATION TIME: 10 MINUTES

1 Using a sharp knife, slice off just enough of one end of the melon to permit the melon to stand upright. Slice the other end down about 1 inch, or until the seeds are exposed.

2 Scoop out the seeds and discard. Cut the melon into 4 equal-sized rings and place each on a small serving dish.

3 Mix the Lemony Yogurt Cheese Spread with the blueberries and place several dollops in the center of each melon ring.

4 Sprinkle each ring with chopped walnuts. Serve immediately.

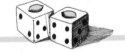

TAKE A CHANCE:

- Mix the yogurt cheese spread with other fresh berries.
- Sprinkle coconut on top.
- Mix the berries with whipped cream cheese and either add a bit of grated lemon zest or squeeze a lemon over the fruit before serving.

Lemonaid

Lemons bring a breath of fresh air and the fragrance of a summer's day into the home no matter what time of year it is.

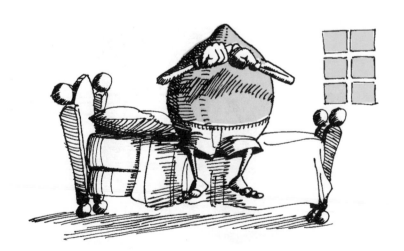

Spicy Applesauce

Good any time of the day, applesauce is easy to make, and our version contains the tart goodness of lemon. Try spooning this over your morning oatmeal.

1 cup water

4 large tart cooking apples, peeled, cored, and quartered

grated zest and juice of 1 medium lemon

$\frac{1}{2}$ teaspoon ground cinnamon

$\frac{1}{8}$ teaspoon ground nutmeg

$\frac{1}{2}$ cup dark raisins (optional)

SERVES: 4   PREPARATION TIME: 30 MINUTES

1 Place the water and apples in a large saucepan and bring to a boil over high heat. Lower the heat to medium, add the lemon juice, and simmer until the apples are tender, about 10 minutes, stirring occasionally.

2 Place the contents of the saucepan in a blender or food processor, and pulse until smooth, working in batches if necessary.

3 Return the applesauce to the pan, add the remaining ingredients, and stir to blend. Simmer for 5 to 10 minutes, or until the spices are incorporated and the raisins are plump. Serve warm or cold.

TAKE A CHANCE:

- Sweeten with a little honey.

- Use red-skinned apples and leave their peels on while cooking. Remove and discard the peel before blending. This will give the applesauce a reddish tinge.

- Leave the applesauce in chunks. Add the remaining ingredients after the apples are tender and simmer until done.

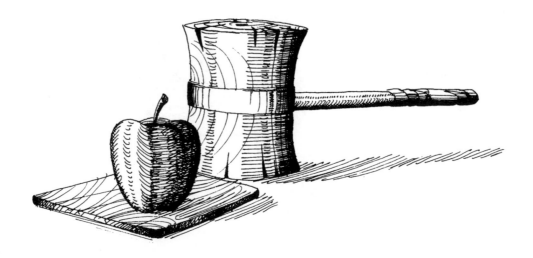

Lemon Spice Fruit Compote

Hot spicy fruit with the fresh taste of lemon is a special treat on a cold morning.

grated zest and juice of 1 medium lemon

1 cup water

$\frac{1}{4}$ cup apple juice concentrate

1 small cinnamon stick

3 apples, peeled, cored, and cut into thick slices

2 pears, peeled, cored, and cut into thick slices

2 peaches, skinned, pitted, and cut into thick slices

$\frac{1}{2}$ cup dark raisins

$\frac{1}{2}$ teaspoon ground cinnamon

SERVES: 4　PREPARATION TIME: 30 MINUTES

1 Place the lemon zest, lemon juice, water, apple juice concentrate, and cinnamon stick in a large pot and bring to a boil over high heat. Lower the heat to medium and simmer for 5 minutes.

2 Discard the cinnamon stick and add the fruit. Simmer for 10 to 15 minutes, or until the fruit is softened.

3 Sprinkle the compote with the ground cinnamon and serve warm.

Note From a Healthy Lemon:

For a special treat in recipes calling for ground cinnamon, grate a cinnamon stick on a hand grater instead of using commercially ground cinnamon. It takes a few minutes to do, but the taste is much more pungent than that of ground cinnamon from a can.

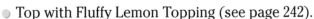

TAKE A CHANCE:

- Top with Fluffy Lemon Topping (see page 242).
- Serve over ice cream or pudding.
- Use fresh berries instead of the apples, pears, and peaches, and reduce the cooking time for the fruit to 3 to 5 minutes.

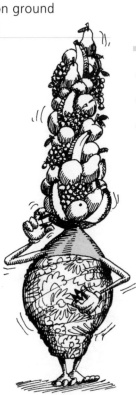

*L*emon Biscuits

*F*resh biscuits hot from the oven go hand-in-hand with breakfast. But don't limit yourself to breakfast. These biscuits make a great addition to any meal.

1 cup unbleached white flour

1 cup whole wheat pastry flour

1 tablespoon baking powder

$\frac{1}{4}$ cup safflower oil

grated zest of 1 medium lemon

$\frac{2}{3}$ cup soymilk

YIELD: 18 BISCUITS   PREPARATION TIME: 45 MINUTES

1 Place the dry ingredients in a large bowl and mix. Stir in the oil until the mixture resembles coarse crumbs. Add the lemon zest and soymilk, and mix just until a soft dough forms.

2 On a lightly floured surface, knead the dough 6 to 8 times. Roll the dough with a lightly floured rolling pin to form a ½-inch-thick sheet.

3 With a floured biscuit cutter or the rim of a 2-inch glass, cut out 18 biscuits. Use a spatula to place the biscuits 1 inch apart on an ungreased cookie sheet and bake in a 450°F oven for 12 to 15 minutes, or until golden brown. Serve immediately.

TAKE A CHANCE:

● Use ½ teaspoon dried lemon thyme instead of the zest.

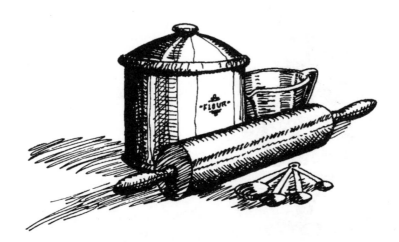

Zesty Breakfast Scones

These scones are very easy to make and satisfying to eat.

2 teaspoons grated lemon zest

1 cup currants

1 cup unbleached white flour

1 cup whole wheat flour

1 teaspoon baking soda

6 tablespoons malt powder

½ cup light sesame or safflower oil

2 medium eggs

¼ cup soymilk

SERVES: 4   PREPARATION TIME: 30 MINUTES

1 Place the lemon zest and currants in a large bowl and mix well. Add the dry ingredients and mix. Add the oil and mix until the dough resembles coarse meal. Add the eggs and soymilk, and combine just until mixed.

2 Divide the dough into two equal portions. Gently pat each portion into a ½-inch-thick circle on a lightly greased cookie sheet. Using a knife, score each circle into 6 wedges, deeply indenting the dough.

3 Bake in a 400°F oven for 12 to 15 minutes, or until brown.

4 Cool for 10 minutes, cut into wedges, and serve.

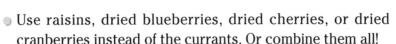

TAKE A CHANCE:

- Use raisins, dried blueberries, dried cherries, or dried cranberries instead of the currants. Or combine them all!

- Spread the warm scones with the curd from Tart Lemon Tartletts (see page 212).

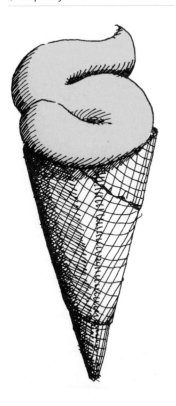

*L*emon Yogurt Muffins

*hese are great first thing in
the morning, warm out of
the oven with a nice tang of
lemon.*

grated zest of 1 medium
lemon

1 large egg

1 cup lemon-flavored
nonfat yogurt

¼ cup soymilk

¼ cup light sesame or
safflower oil

1¼ cups unbleached white
flour

1¼ cups whole wheat
pastry flour

¼ cup date sugar

1 tablespoon baking powder

YIELD: 12 MUFFINS   PREPARATION TIME: 30 MINUTES

1 Stir together the lemon zest, egg, yogurt, soymilk, and oil
in a large mixing bowl. Add both of the flours, the date
sugar, and the baking powder, mixing just until the flour is
moistened. Do not overmix.

2 Fill greased muffin cups ⅔ full and bake in a 400°F oven for
20 minutes, or until a toothpick inserted in the center of a
muffin comes out clean.

3 Immediately remove the muffins from the pan and cool for
5 minutes before serving.

TAKE A CHANCE:

● Add ½ cup blueberries or cranberries.

● Drizzle with Lemon Cinnamon Glaze (see page 240).

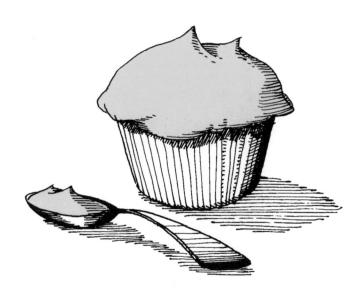

Cranberry Breakfast Bread

This bread is wonderful any time of the day, although it doesn't often make it past the breakfast table. Make several loaves at once and freeze for a quick treat. Freeze some fresh cranberries in the fall and enjoy this breakfast bread all year long.

grated zest of 1 medium lemon

2 tablespoons lemon juice

1½ cups whole cranberries, coarsely chopped

¼ cup malt powder

3 cups whole wheat pastry flour

4 teaspoons baking powder

1 large egg

1½ cups soymilk

2 tablespoons safflower oil

YIELD: 1 LOAF   PREPARATION TIME: 1½ HOURS

1 Place the lemon zest, lemon juice, cranberries, and 2 tablespoons of the malt powder in a small bowl, mix, and set aside.

2 Combine the flour, baking powder, and remaining malt powder in a large bowl. Add the egg, soymilk, and oil, and stir. Add the cranberry mixture and stir just until the cranberries are incorporated into the batter. The batter will be slightly stiff.

3 Pour the batter into a lightly greased 9-x-5-inch loaf pan and bake in a 350°F oven for 1 hour, or until a toothpick inserted in the center of the bread comes out clean.

4 Remove the pan from the oven and allow the bread to cool in the pan for 10 minutes. Run a knife around the sides of the pan to loosen the bread in the pan and transfer it to a serving plate. Serve warm or at room temperature.

Note From a Healthy Lemon:

Frozen cranberries do not need to be thawed before being added to the recipe.

TAKE A CHANCE:

- Serve with Lemony Yogurt Cheese Spread (see page 236).
- Reduce the cranberries to 1 cup and add ½ cup chopped walnuts.

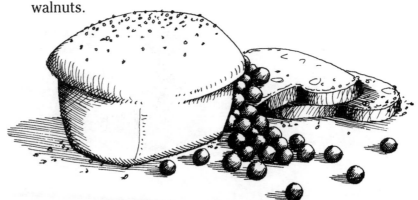

Honey-Glazed Lemon Walnut Bread

The perfect accompaniment to a special breakfast, this loaf is also satisfying by itself.

Bread

grated zest of 1 medium lemon

$\frac{1}{2}$ cup soymilk

3 tablespoons safflower oil

2 tablespoons Sucanat

2 large eggs

$1\frac{1}{2}$ cups whole wheat pastry flour

1 teaspoon baking powder

$\frac{1}{4}$ cup chopped walnuts

Glaze

juice of 1 medium lemon

2 tablespoons honey

YIELD: 1 LOAF   PREPARATION TIME: 1½ HOURS

1 To make the bread, place the lemon zest and the soymilk in a large bowl and mix. Stir in the oil and Sucanat. Add the eggs one at a time, beating well after each addition. Gradually stir in the flour and baking powder. Stir in the walnuts.

2 Pour the batter into a greased and floured 9-x-5-inch loaf pan and bake in a 350°F oven for 50 to 55 minutes, or until a toothpick inserted in the center of the bread comes out clean. Remove the bread from the oven.

3 To make the glaze, heat the lemon juice and honey in a small saucepan until the honey has dissolved. Slowly pour the mixture over the top of the bread while the bread is still in the pan.

4 Cool the bread completely, remove from the pan, and serve.

TAKE A CHANCE:

● Use Lemon Cinnamon Glaze (see page 240) instead of the Honey Glaze.

● Use pecans instead of the walnuts.

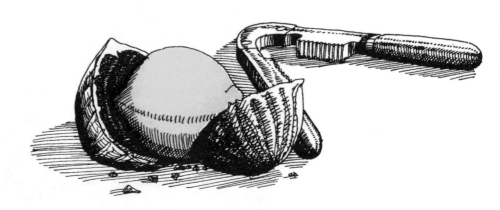

Rise and Shine Lemon Loaf

Rich and moist, this bread has a savory lemon flavor.

grated zest of 1 medium lemon

$\frac{1}{3}$ cup unfiltered apple juice

1 large egg

$\frac{1}{3}$ cup light sesame or safflower oil

$1\frac{1}{4}$ cups whole wheat pastry flour

1 teaspoon baking powder

$\frac{1}{2}$ cup soymilk

YIELD: 1 LOAF   PREPARATION TIME: $1\frac{1}{2}$ HOURS

1 Place the lemon zest, apple juice, egg, and oil in a large bowl, mix, and set aside.

2 Mix the flour and baking powder together in a small bowl and alternately add the flour mixture and the soymilk to the egg mixture, stirring only until the mixture is blended.

3 Pour the batter into a greased and floured 9-x-5-inch loaf pan and bake in a 350°F oven for 55 to 60 minutes, or until a toothpick inserted in the center of the bread comes out clean.

4 Cool completely and serve.

TAKE A CHANCE:

● Add ¼ cup chopped pecans, almonds, or walnuts to the batter.

● Top the loaf with Lemon Cinnamon Glaze (see page 240).

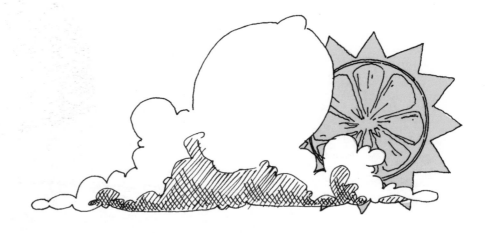

*L*emon Poppy Seed Muffins

*S*parkling with fresh lemon and crunchy with poppy seeds, these muffins won't last past breakfast time.

1 tablespoon lemon juice

grated zest of 1 medium lemon

2 large eggs

$\frac{1}{4}$ cup safflower oil

3 tablespoons date sugar

$\frac{1}{2}$ cup soymilk

$1\frac{1}{4}$ cups unbleached white flour

1 teaspoon baking powder

3 tablespoons poppy seeds

YIELD: 12 MUFFINS   PREPARATION TIME: 30 MINUTES

1 Place the lemon juice, lemon zest, and eggs in a large bowl and mix. Add the oil and date sugar, and mix well. Add the remaining ingredients and stir just until blended.

2 Fill greased and floured muffin cups ¾ full and bake in a 350°F oven for 15 to 20 minutes, or until a toothpick inserted in the center of a muffin comes out clean.

3 Immediately remove the muffins from the pan and cool for 5 minutes before serving.

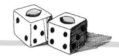

TAKE A CHANCE:

- Top with Lemon Cinnamon Glaze (see page 240).

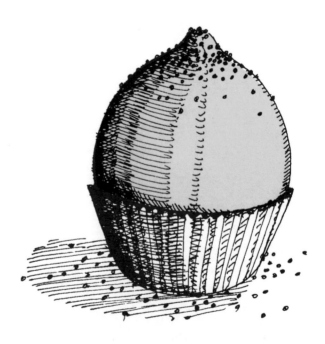

Lemon Loaf Surprise

The surprise is the mixture of lemon with dried cherries. A pleasing combination at breakfast or tea time.

2¾ cups unbleached white flour

1 teaspoon baking powder

¼ teaspoon ground nutmeg

grated zest of 1 medium lemon

1 tablespoon lemon juice

½ cup finely chopped dried cherries

¼ cup melted soy margarine

3 tablespoons apple juice concentrate

1 cup soymilk

1 large egg

YIELD: 1 LOAF   PREPARATION TIME: 1 HOUR

1 Place all the dry ingredients in a large bowl and stir to blend. Add the remaining ingredients and stir just until moistened.

2 Pour the batter into a greased 9-x-5-inch loaf pan and bake in a 350°F oven for 40 to 45 minutes, or until a toothpick inserted in the center of the loaf comes out clean. Cool for 10 minutes and remove from the pan.

3 Slice the loaf and serve immediately.

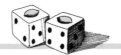

TAKE A CHANCE:

- Top with Lemon Cinnamon Glaze (see page 240).

- Serve with Honey and Lemon Spread (see page 241) or Lemony Yogurt Cheese Spread (see page 236).

- Make the loaf with different dried fruits, such as papaya, mango, or apricot.

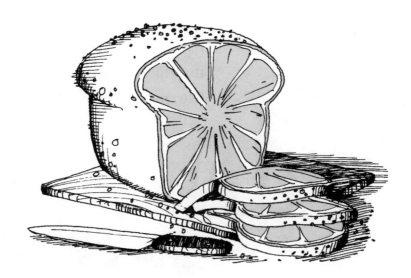

Lemon-Glazed Blueberry Loaf

The lemon-blueberry taste of this moist loaf is delightful.

Loaf

grated zest of 2 medium lemons

$\frac{1}{2}$ cup soymilk

2 large eggs

$\frac{1}{4}$ cup canola oil

2 tablespoons Sucanat

1 cup unbleached white flour

$1\frac{2}{3}$ cups whole wheat pastry flour

2 teaspoons baking powder

$1\frac{1}{2}$ cups blueberries, hulled

Glaze

juice of 1 medium lemon

1 tablespoon date sugar

YIELD: 1 LOAF   PREPARATION TIME: $1\frac{1}{2}$ HOURS

1 To make the loaf, mix the lemon zest, soymilk, eggs, oil, and Sucanat in a large bowl until smooth. Stir in the flours and baking powder, mixing just until the flour is moist. Fold in the blueberries.

2 Pour the batter into a greased 9-x-5-inch loaf pan and bake in a 350°F oven for 1 hour, or until a toothpick inserted in the center of the loaf comes out clean.

3 To make the glaze, combine the lemon juice and date sugar in a small saucepan over high heat, stirring constantly. Continue to cook until the liquid becomes syrupy, 1 to 2 minutes.

4 While the loaf is still in the pan, pour the warm glaze over the loaf and let the loaf remain in the pan for 15 minutes.

5 Transfer the loaf from the pan to a wire rack and cool completely before serving.

TAKE A CHANCE:

- Combine $\frac{1}{3}$ cup chopped walnuts or pecans with the lemon zest.

- Use frozen blueberries instead of the fresh. (You need not thaw the fruit before folding it into the batter.)

- Use cranberries instead of the blueberries.

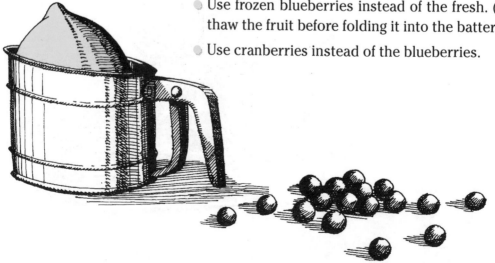

Lemon Sliver Marmalade

This special treat is an excellent way to use up some of those extra lemons. A tablespoon of this summer sunshine will brighten up even the most dreary winter morning.

1 cup thinly sliced lemons, cut into slivers

2 cups water

1 cup date sugar

1 cup concentrated fruit sweetener

YIELD: 1 PINT   PREPARATION TIME: 3 HOURS

1 Place the lemon slivers and the water in a large pot and bring to a boil over high heat. Continue boiling until the lemons are tender. Remove the pot from the heat and stir in the date sugar and concentrated fruit sweetener.

2 Transfer 2 cups of the lemon mixture to a saucepan and cook for 10 to 15 minutes, or until the mixture thickens. Pour into hot sterile jars and cover. Repeat this process with the remaining mixture. Allow the jars to cool at room temperature for 1 hour, then refrigerate until cold.

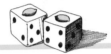

TAKE A CHANCE:

● Use a mixture of half lemons and half oranges.

Lemonaid

Commercially made pectin for jellies and jams comes from the pith of the lemon.

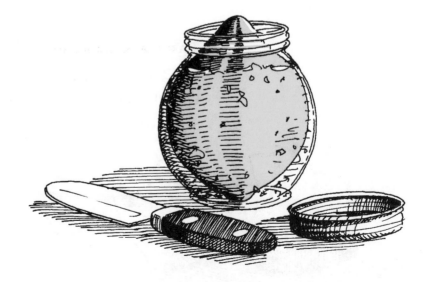

Citrus Omelet With a Slice of Sunshine Salad

This eye opener will definitely chase away those early or late morning blues.

8 large eggs

$\frac{1}{4}$ cup soymilk

$\frac{1}{2}$ teaspoon Lemon Pepper (see page 227)

$\frac{1}{4}$ cup soy margarine

grated zest of 1 medium lemon

grated zest of 1 large orange

1 tablespoon chopped fresh chives

A Slice of Sunshine Salad (see page 62)

SERVES: 4   PREPARATION TIME: 20 MINUTES

1 Place 2 of the eggs, 1 tablespoon of the soymilk, and a sprinkling of the Lemon Pepper in a small bowl and beat with a wire whisk.

2 Melt 1 tablespoon of the soy margarine in an omelet pan or small skillet, and heat until very hot but not brown.

3 Pour the beaten eggs into the heated pan and rapidly slide the skillet back and forth over the burner. At the same time, tilt the pan so the egg covers the entire bottom of the skillet. Cook just until the bottom is set, then remove from the heat.

4 Add a portion of the grated lemon and orange zest to the third of the omelet closest to you. Run a fork around the edges of the omelet to loosen it from the pan and fold the zest-covered part of the omelet toward the center. Slide the omelet out of the pan onto a heated serving dish and fold the top third over the center of the omelet. Repeat the steps with the remaining eggs to make 3 more omelets.

5 Sprinkle the omelets with the chives and serve immediately with A Slice of Sunshine Salad.

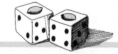

TAKE A CHANCE:

- Fold 1 tablespoon diced mushrooms inside the omelet.
- Cook the omelet in Mock Lemon Butter (see page 235).
- Serve with Fresh Lemony Salsa (see page 59).

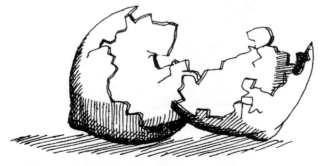

Egg Burritos With Fresh Lemony Salsa

There is no such thing as plain scrambled eggs when tortillas and salsa are nearby. Olé!

6 large eggs

2 tablespoons soymilk

½ teaspoon Lemon Pepper (see page 227)

2 teaspoons soy margarine

4 organic whole wheat tortillas, 12 inches each, warmed

½ cup Fresh Lemony Salsa (see page 59)

SERVES: 4   PREPARATION TIME: 10 MINUTES

1 Place the eggs, soymilk, and Lemon Pepper in a small bowl and whisk together.

2 Melt the margarine in a large skillet. Add the egg mixture and cook over medium heat, stirring constantly, until the eggs are done.

3 Divide the eggs evenly among the tortillas and add 1 tablespoon of salsa to each. Fold in the sides of the tortillas and roll the burritos closed.

4 Serve immediately with additional salsa on the side.

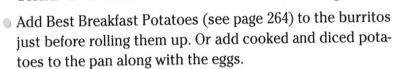

TAKE A CHANCE:

- Add Best Breakfast Potatoes (see page 264) to the burritos just before rolling them up. Or add cooked and diced potatoes to the pan along with the eggs.

- Add ¼ cup coarsely chopped mushrooms to the margarine and sauté for 1 minute before adding the eggs.

- Omit the salsa and tortillas, and serve the eggs with Lemony Hollandaise Sauce (see page 230).

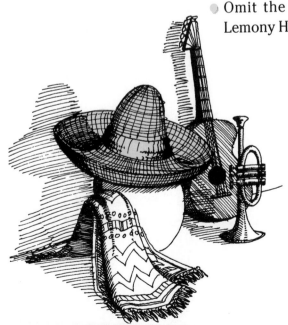

*B*est Breakfast Potatoes

Your mouth will think it has gone on vacation with these wonderful home-fried potatoes. Make extra, because it's very hard to keep your fingers out of the pan "just to see if they're done."

2 tablespoons light sesame or safflower oil

1 medium onion, thinly sliced and separated into rings

4 large potatoes, thinly sliced

$\frac{1}{2}$ teaspoon paprika

1 teaspoon Lemon Pepper (see page 227)

SERVES: 4   PREPARATION TIME: 45 MINUTES

1 Heat the oil in a large skillet and sauté the onion over high heat for 3 minutes, stirring constantly. Add the potatoes and paprika, and sauté for 2 minutes, turning continuously until the potatoes are coated with oil. Reduce the heat to medium, cover the pan, and cook until the potatoes are done, about 30 minutes, stirring occasionally.

2 Add the Lemon Pepper, toss, and serve immediately.

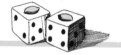

TAKE A CHANCE:

- Add ½ cup diced red or green bell pepper to the potatoes before cooking.

- Use cayenne pepper instead of the paprika.

- Try these potatoes in Egg Burritos With Fresh Lemony Salsa (see page 263).

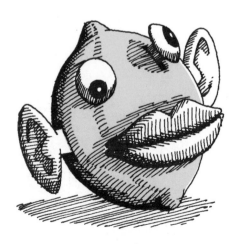

*L*imon Pancake à Deux

While this recipe makes enough for a cozy breakfast for two under the lemon tree, it can easily be adjusted to serve large crowds of lemon lovers.

½ cup soymilk

2 large eggs

½ cup oat flour

grated zest and juice of 1 medium lemon

1 tablespoon melted soy margarine

1 medium lemon, cut into wedges

SERVES: 2   PREPARATION TIME: 20 MINUTES

1 Place the soymilk and eggs in a large bowl and mix. Slowly add the flour, stirring constantly, until the batter is smooth. Stir in the lemon zest and juice.

2 Coat an 8-inch skillet with the melted margarine and add the batter. Bake in a 475°F oven for 10 to 12 minutes, or until the pancake is puffed and golden brown.

3 Divide the pancake into portions and transfer to individual plates. Garnish with the lemon wedges and serve immediately.

TAKE A CHANCE:

● Serve with Honey and Lemon Spread (see page 241) or Lemon Fruit Syrup (see page 244).

● Top with Berry, Berry Lemony (see page 248).

● Use a combination of grated lemon and orange zest.

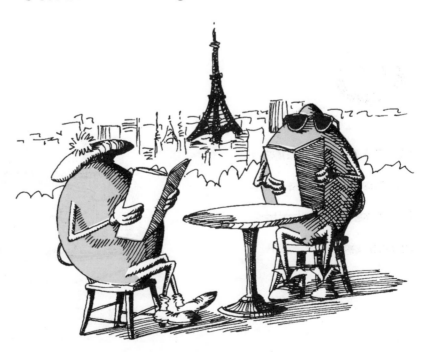

Buckwheat Pancakes With Lemon Fruit Syrup

These pancakes are a bright and sunny morning treat.

2 large eggs

2 tablespoons light sesame or safflower oil

2 cups soymilk

1 cup unbleached white flour

1 cup buckwheat flour

2 teaspoons baking powder

1 tablespoon honey

1 tablespoon melted soy margarine

grated zest of 2 medium lemons

Lemon Fruit Syrup (see page 244)

SERVES: 4   PREPARATION TIME: 20 MINUTES

1 Place the eggs, oil, and soymilk in a large bowl and whisk together. Add the flours, baking powder, and honey, and continue whisking until the batter is smooth.

2 Coat a hot griddle with the melted margarine and pour the batter onto the griddle in 4-inch rounds. Turn the pancakes with a spatula when the pancakes puff and bubbles form. Cook the pancakes on the other side until browned.

3 Transfer the pancakes to serving plates, garnish with the grated lemon zest, and serve immediately with the Lemon Fruit Syrup.

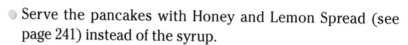

TAKE A CHANCE:

- Serve the pancakes with Honey and Lemon Spread (see page 241) instead of the syrup.

- Mix the lemon zest into the pancake batter.

Lemonaid

Drying concentrates the oils in the zest, but fresh zest is still better in recipes.

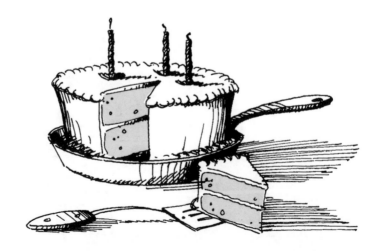

Lighter-Than-Air Lemon Waffles

These feather-light waffles are made to order for anyone with a cholesterol problem or anyone who is trying hard to keep that youthful figure.

2 tablespoons lemon juice

2 cups soymilk

1 cup oat bran

1 cup unbleached white flour

2 teaspoons baking powder

3 tablespoons canola oil

grated zest of 1 medium lemon

4 large egg whites

S ERVES : 4   P REPARATION T IME : 30 MINUTES

1 Place the lemon juice and soymilk in a small bowl and set aside for 5 minutes.

2 Place the oat bran, flour, and baking powder in a large bowl and mix. Add the soymilk and oil, and stir until the batter is smooth. Stir in the grated lemon zest.

3 In a small mixing bowl, beat the egg whites with an electric mixer until stiff. Fold the eggs into the batter.

4 For each waffle, pour some batter from a cup onto the middle of a heated waffle iron and cook for 5 minutes, or until the iron stops steaming and the waffle is golden brown.

5 Transfer to a serving plate and serve immediately.

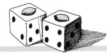

T AKE A C HANCE :

● Use 1 cup oat flour instead of the oat bran.

● Top with Mock Lemon Butter (see page 235) or Lemon Fruit Syrup (see page 244). Or try Berry, Berry Lemony (see page 248) or Honey and Lemon Spread (see page 241).

Lemonaid

For centuries, lemon verbena has been a favorite ingredient in colognes and sachets.

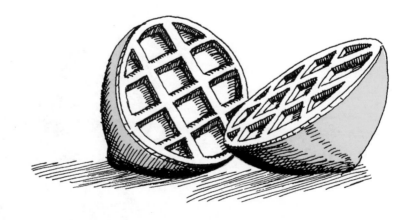

*L*emon French Toast

*F*rench toast is always such a treat—but ours has a special lemony secret.

2 tablespoons Mock Lemon Butter (see page 235)

grated zest and juice of 1 medium lemon

1 large egg

1½ cups soymilk

1 teaspoon date sugar

8 slices whole wheat bread

¼ teaspoon ground cinnamon

SERVES: 4   PREPARATION TIME: 20 MINUTES

1 Melt the Mock Lemon Butter on a large griddle.

2 Place the lemon zest, lemon juice, egg, soymilk, and date sugar in a large bowl and beat until smooth. Dip the bread slices in the egg mixture until saturated and place on the griddle. Sauté the slices 4 to 5 minutes over medium-high heat on each side, or until golden brown.

3 Transfer the French toast to warmed plates, sprinkle with the ground cinnamon, and serve immediately.

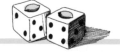

TAKE A CHANCE:

● Place the egg-dipped bread slices on a greased baking sheet and bake in a 500°F oven for 8 minutes on each side.

● Top with Honey and Lemon Spread (see page 241) or Lemon Fruit Syrup (see page 244).

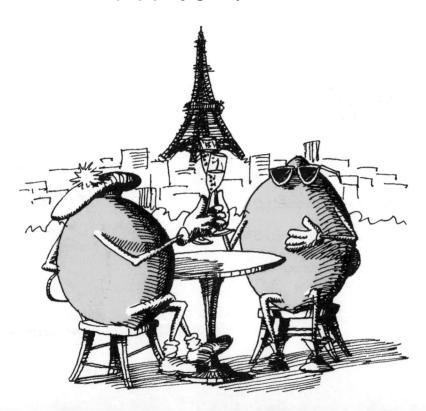

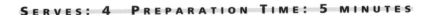
Lemon-Kissed Oatmeal

When the idea for this book was first being batted around, the joke was that about the only thing you couldn't put lemon on was oatmeal. Wrong! That opinion was revised after this dish was sampled.

2⅔ cups water

1⅓ cups rolled oats

2 teaspoons grated lemon zest

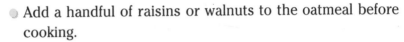

SERVES: 4   PREPARATION TIME: 5 MINUTES

1 In a small saucepan, bring the water to a boil over high heat. Add the oats slowly, stirring constantly. Reduce the heat to medium and cook for 2 minutes, or until thickened, stirring constantly.

2 Sprinkle the oatmeal with the lemon zest and serve immediately.

TAKE A CHANCE:

- Add a handful of raisins or walnuts to the oatmeal before cooking.
- Add ¼ teaspoon cinnamon to the cereal before cooking.
- Serve with Spicy Applesauce (see page 250).

Lemonaid

No kitchen is complete without lemons tucked away somewhere.

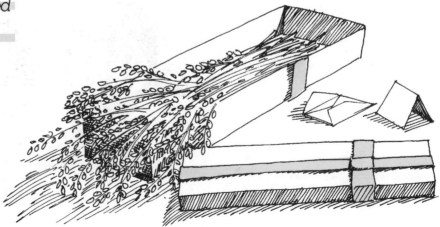

Farewell, but Not Goodbye

All too soon, this concludes our exploration of the lemon and its roles. Keep experimenting, and we're sure you'll find many more lemony delights than we have been able to include in this volume. We wish you peace and happiness as you discover that a lemon in your life is a very good thing.

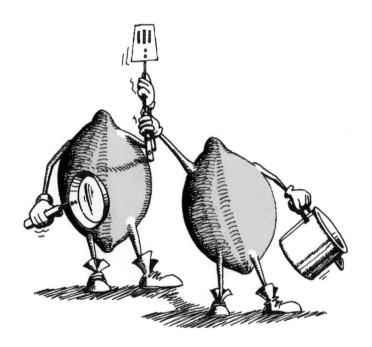

Index